WAR AND HEALTH

ANTHROPOLOGIES OF AMERICAN MEDICINE:
CULTURE, POWER, AND PRACTICE

General Editors: Paul Brodwin, Michele Rivkin-Fish, and Susan Shaw

Transnational Reproduction: Race, Kinship, and Commercial Surrogacy in India
Daisy Deomampo

Unequal Coverage: The Experience of Health Care Reform in the United States
Edited by Jessica Mulligan and Heide Castañeda

Inequalities of Aging: Paradoxes of Independence in American Home Care
Elana D. Buch

The New American Servitude: Political Belonging among African Immigrant Home Care Workers
Cati Coe

Reproductive Injustice: Racism, Pregnancy, and Premature Birth
Dána-Ain Davis

War and Health: The Medical Consequences of the Wars in Iraq and Afghanistan
Edited by Catherine Lutz and Andrea Mazzarino

War and Health

The Medical Consequences of the Wars in Iraq and Afghanistan

EDITED BY

Catherine Lutz and Andrea Mazzarino

NEW YORK UNIVERSITY PRESS
New York

NEW YORK UNIVERSITY PRESS
New York
www.nyupress.org

© 2019 by New York University

All rights reserved

References to Internet websites (URLs) were accurate at the time of writing. Neither the author nor New York University Press is responsible for URLs that may have expired or changed since the manuscript was prepared.

Library of Congress Cataloging-in-Publication Data
Names: Lutz, Catherine, editor. | Mazzarino, Andrea, editor.
Title: War and health : the medical consequences of the wars in Iraq and Afghanistan / edited by Catherine Lutz and Andrea Mazzarino.
Other titles: Anthropologies of American medicine.
Description: New York : New York University Press, 2019. | Series: Anthropologies of american medicine : culture, power, and practice | Includes bibliographical references and index.
Identifiers: LCCN 2018060119 | ISBN 9781479875962 (cl : alk. paper) | ISBN 9781479894611 (pb : alk. paper)
Subjects: LCSH: Afghan War, 2001-   —Health aspects. | Iraq War, 2003–2011—Health aspects. | Public health—Afghanistan—History—21st century. | Public health—Pakistan—History—21st century. | Public health—Iraq—History—21st century.
Classification: LCC RA541.A3 W37 2019 | DDC 362.109581—dc23
LC record available at https://lccn.loc.gov/2018060119

New York University Press books are printed on acid-free paper, and their binding materials are chosen for strength and durability. We strive to use environmentally responsible suppliers and materials to the greatest extent possible in publishing our books.

Manufactured in the United States of America

10 9 8 7 6 5 4 3 2 1

Also available as an ebook

We dedicate this book to the people who have borne the brunt of the wars in Afghanistan, Iraq, and Pakistan—namely, civilians and uniformed forces living in the war zones, and US veterans and their families. We hope that the story we tell pushes governments one step closer to understanding the costs of war on health, and consequently, to creating more peaceful and humane public policies.

We also thank the growing team of the Costs of War Project, who include scholars, physicians, and activists from around the world who do brave and important work telling the story of how these wars devastate people and their communities.

CONTENTS

Introduction: The Health Consequences of War *Andrea Mazzarino, Marcia C. Inhorn, and Catherine Lutz*	1

PART I. AFGHANISTAN AND PAKISTAN

1. Childbirth in the Context of Conflict in Afghanistan *Kylea Laina Liese*	41
2. Drone Strikes and Vaccination Campaigns: How the War on Terror Helps Sustain Polio in Afghanistan and Pakistan *Svea Closser and Noah Coburn*	57
3. Remaining Undone: Heroin in the Time of Serial War *Anila Daulatzai*	73
4. Dignity under Extreme Duress: The Moral and Emotional Landscape of Local Humanitarian Workers in the Afghan-Pakistan Border Areas *Patricia Omidian and Catherine Panter-Brick*	90

PART II. IRAQ

5. War and the Public Health Disaster in Iraq *Scott Harding and Kathryn Libal*	111
6. The Political Capital of War Wounds *Ghassan Soleiman Abu-Sittah*	137
7. Iraqis' Cancer Itineraries: War, Medical Travel, and Therapeutic Geographies *Mac Skelton*	152
8. War and Its Consequences for Cancer Trends and Services in Iraq *Layth Mula-Hussain*	172

PART III. UNITED STATES

9. Imagining Military Suicide 191
   Ken MacLeish

10. Afterwar Work for Life 210
    Zoë H. Wool

11. "It's Not Okay": War's Toll on Health Brought Home to Communities and Environments 231
    Jean Scandlyn and Sarah Hautzinger

Appendix: The Body Count 255
   Neta Crawford

About the Editors 259

About the Contributors 261

Index 265

Introduction

The Health Consequences of War

ANDREA MAZZARINO, MARCIA C. INHORN, AND
CATHERINE LUTZ

For those of us who have never lived through a war, it is hard to imagine what it would be like—the bombings, sniper fire, unexploded ordnance, abductions and imprisonment, house raids, torture, rape, and surviving families' flight from all of it. Beyond the bombs and bullets, war brings privation: loss of access to food, water, and electricity; bombed out hospitals, schools, and many other institutions of human welfare and community; and loss of trust and emotional equanimity. These are the kinds of horrors that war inflicts on human beings, both combatants and civilians. Indeed, in the twentieth century, it is estimated that 45 million combatants and 62 million civilians died as a result of war—not only as a result of its violence, but when diseases and hunger that war spawned took even more lives than did battlefield injuries (Ostrach and Singer 2013).

The carnage does not show signs of abating. Global data compiled by the Geneva Declaration on Armed Violence and Development shows that the number of conflict-related deaths increased by 27 percent between the periods 2004–2009 and 2007–2012 (Geneva Declaration Secretariat 2015, 12, 2).

Standing out for its global scope, its longevity, and the constantly morphing cast of actors and geographic locations in which it has occurred is the US-led "war on terror" initiated after the September 11, 2001 attacks on New York City and Washington, DC. In Afghanistan, Iraq, and Pakistan, where the United States has waged wars for more than a decade and a half, the devastation affecting local civilians and combatants is seldom covered by the US press in detail or in ways that go beyond the image of the rubble or twisted metal in a bombing's aftermath. These wars and their human health costs are the cases examined in this volume. What our authors show, above all else, is that the shock waves war sends through the human body extend through and beyond it in time and context more than is typically understood. The assaults of war are not only the kinetic ones with which we are most familiar, but the health degradation that occurs as an indirect result of war and that continues long after a war is putatively over. As has been shown most vividly by Johnston and colleagues (2007) in their studies of the health effects of nuclear testing, the legacy of war and war preparation is found in their shaping of both physical being and sociocultural identity. The harms can be invisible, as with radioactive materials' or other war toxins' corrosive effects on the communities in which weapons are made or tested, and they can extend decades forward in time as injuries are compounded by age or neglect, or social orders are remade by diaspora and economic collapse that leave whole regions with inadequate healthcare or food supplies. As Johnston (2007) and Barker (2004) have also demonstrated, the communities under the bombs are often the least powerful from the start of hostilities, and their ability to seek care for their war injuries and other losses is correspondingly constrained.

The impetus for this book began in 2010, when Catherine Lutz and Andrea Mazzarino set out, along with Boston University political scientist Neta Crawford, to tell as full as possible a story about the consequences that ensued when the United States responded with military force to the September 11, 2001 attacks. Focusing on the wars in Afghanistan, Iraq, and Pakistan, we sought to highlight more than their mounting costs in dollars: We foregrounded lives lost, damaged, and disrupted, including among civilians in those war zones, as well as US uniformed service members, contractors, and other combatants. We assembled a team of more than thirty social scientists, human rights activists, and physicians with expertise in the broad range of war's impact and created a public website (www.costsofwar.org) embedded with their reports and graphics to illustrate the many human and material costs exacted by those wars. That information was disseminated as the work of the Costs of War Project beginning in June 2011 and provided journalists and the general public with more reliable information as they reflected on the tenth anniversary of the 9/11 attacks later that year.

We expanded our coverage to include the United States' ongoing counterterrorism operations in Yemen since 2002, consisting of Special Forces operations, air strikes, and drone attacks and support for ground combat in the war against the Islamic State in Syria and northern Iraq. The Project, now more than forty-five researchers strong, continues to generate reports and press coverage of, and political attention to, the findings on many aspects of the wars' consequences, including damage to human health.

To 2018, it is estimated that at least 480,000 people had been killed by violence in the Afghanistan, Iraq, and Pakistan wars (see appendix; Crawford 2018c). While indirect deaths are even more difficult than direct deaths to enumerate, an estimated additional at least 1 million people have likely died as an indirect result of the wars, that is, they have died from illnesses, injuries, and malnutrition that would not have occurred without the wars' economic, social, and healthcare disruptions or reallocation of resources to deal with the directly injured. All told then, in Iraq, Afghanistan, and Pakistan, there have been well over a million and a half civilians and combatants killed to date (Costs of War Project 2017).

It is the large number of indirect deaths from these wars (as well as the failure of most of the very large literature on war to focus on its concrete and multifarious health effects rather than simply its strategic or social dimensions) that prompted our concentration on their varied health consequences for civilians in the war zones, as well as for active-duty US service members and veterans and for other fighting forces. It struck us that war held far-reaching consequences for families, communities, and healthcare systems even in the United States with its sophisticated healthcare infrastructure, and with many more consequences in Iraq with its once relatively developed and regionally eminent system, and in Afghanistan and Pakistan, where poverty and underinvestment in public services have together made healthcare less advanced and accessible. So too in light of sequential wars in both countries: in Iraq since the war with Iran from 1980–88, followed by the 1991 Gulf War, followed by the sanctions war from 1991 to 2003, and in Afghanistan a variety of conflicts since the Soviet invasion of 1979 straight through to the US 2001 invasion. War creates an amalgam of health crises that are global in scale. We saw the need to paint a picture of those crises and to expose some of their structural underpinnings.

This volume seeks to inform the general public as well as scholars and students in college classrooms of the many health costs of these wars, both on the battlefield, and elsewhere—in hospitals, homes, and refugee camps; and both during combat and in the years following, as communities struggle to live normal lives despite decimated social services, ongoing illness and disability, and the loss of loved ones.

The authors of our chapters are, in the main, anthropologists who have conducted ethnographic fieldwork in order to reach their conclusions. In-depth, long-term, and culturally and historically informed study of communities in Iraq, Afghanistan, Pakistan, and the United States is an irreplaceable methodology for understanding the world from the point of view of those whose words and experiences are usually missing when Americans speak of war. Unfortunately, there is a very small number of courageous scholars who have done the work of extended research in these (or other) war zones. As a result, this book's coverage of many of the health problems that accompany these wars is not at all comprehensive. This introduction attempts to provide an overview of the problem and, en route, to suggest what other kinds of field research desperately need to be done. That includes research to give a richer sense of how civilian physical health and care regimes are affected in migrant camps and where people shelter in place; how children's physical health is affected by the distinct exposures afforded by their play and curiosity; what the pathways of disease are from destroyed electrical power stations to such unexpected occurrences as increased rates of electrocution or falls as people cope with damaged urban infrastructure; better understanding of the fear of contamination brought by war and its weapons and attempts to cope; the ideologies, politics, and profit streams involved in the reconstruction of healthcare systems; and the larger systemic effects of allocating resources to war rather than to social welfare, with ethnographically discoverable cases and processes of morbidity and mortality that result.

Above all, we aim to provide an alternative portrait of war that departs from frequent but limited media images of bombing raids seen from above or of US veterans persevering through their injuries. Wars for those living through them are disturbing, chaotic, and, as this volume shows, unhealthy in innumerable and long-lasting ways. Understanding these ripple effects of war and, more broadly, changing patterns of lethal violence worldwide, is vital to informing public policies aimed at reducing levels of deadly violence (Geneva Declaration Secretariat 2015, 2).

The Syndemics of War

War damages human health through multiple routes, both during and after conflict. The health consequences of war tend to co-occur. Problems such as malnutrition and infectious disease often go hand in hand during wartime, because food shortages and unsanitary living conditions take their toll on human populations, especially those fleeing to makeshift refugee camps. Thus, for every individual who died violently in the wars fought around the world between 2004 and 2007 (estimated at around 600,000 people), another four are estimated to have died from war-related disease and malnutrition (Geneva Declaration Secretariat 2008). That ratio is highly variable, with it often being lower where preexisting impoverished conditions, as in Afghanistan, make the destruction of infrastructure less consequential (the negative health effects of that lack already being reflected in health statistics) and higher in wealthier societies, like Iraq. It is also highly variable depending on whether attacks on civilians and civilian infrastructure are avoided or perpetrated; in the first Gulf War, the United States and its allies destroyed the majority of the Baghdad area's electrical system, and the ripple effects of that destruction resulted in an estimated thirty times more civilian deaths—70,000–90,000 deaths—than did direct war violence (Crawford 2016, 2018b). It also matters whether people continue to live within partially destroyed infrastructure. So it was that injury from falls rose significantly in Iraq as people moved to unrailed rooftops to spend hot days without air-conditioning or fell in the unsafe conditions of a blast-damaged home (Lafta et al. 2015).

Medical anthropologists Bayla Ostrach and Merrill Singer (2013) call these synergistic interactions of war-related morbidity and mortality the "syndemics of war." As they note: "War, by causing physical and emotional trauma in populations, destroying healthcare systems and social infrastructure, despoiling the environment, intentionally or unintentionally causing or exacerbating food insecurity and malnutrition, creating refugee populations, and spreading infections (e.g. through the movement of troops, dislocation of civilian populations, changes in the environment) promotes the development of syndemics" (Ostrach and Singer 2013, 257).

The syndemics of war touch the lives of those who actually fight wars (i.e., combatants, including soldiers, militia members, and increasingly, military contractors); refugees and internally displaced persons; healthcare professionals; and those civilians in or fleeing the war zones.

Physical Costs

War kills people directly and immediately, as well as indirectly and in the aftermath of battle, with indirect casualties far exceeding direct casualties. For example, in 1999, the WHO estimated that 269,000 people around the world died from the direct effects of war; that same year, based on a cross-national analysis of casualty data on both civil and international wars, Ghobarah, Huth, and Russett (2004) estimate that an additional 15 million people died or became disabled as a result of civil wars fought between 1991 and 1997. They emphasize that bombs and bullets are not the only causes of death in war, and soldiers not their primary victims. In fact, infectious diseases are hypothesized to be the principal cause of indirect deaths from war (Ostrach and Singer 2013): War decimates infrastructure including water pipes and healthcare systems, contributes to the breakdown of social norms that make sexual assault less likely, and leads to food insecurity and malnutrition. All of these factors raise the incidence of infectious diseases already existing in the population (e.g., malaria, tuberculosis, respiratory infections, diarrheal disease, polio), and introduce new infectious diseases (e.g., measles, human papilloma virus, HIV/AIDS, and cervical cancer).

Changes in social norms during wartime affect public health in ways that cannot always be predicted. The chapter by medical anthropologists Svea Closser and Noah Coburn shows how polio vaccination campaigns in the Pakistani-Afghan borderlands run up against serious roadblocks in a climate of fear and mistrust toward Americans amidst the ongoing US drone war. A Pakistani grandfather asked, "America drops bombs on us Muslims but then says they are sending vaccines to help us?" His question makes bitter sense in a region of ongoing conflict, the Pakistani government's long-term neglect of other forms of health provision, and local mistrust following the CIA's fake vaccination campaign in the lead-up to the 2011 Osama bin Laden assassination. We gain a rare glimpse into how these communities' resistance to public health programs that seem benevolent on their face are actually adaptive responses to never-ending violence.

Millions of people must also adapt by fleeing violence, leading to large populations of refugees (those who are forced to flee across international borders), as well as Internally Displaced Persons (IDPs, or those who are forced to flee to a different location within the country). As of 2015, more than 60 million people around the world were forcibly displaced by armed conflict and natural disasters. These are the highest levels of displacement on record, according to the United Nations High Commissioner for Refugees (Edwards 2016). One-half of the world's refugees that year were children. Refugee and IDP populations tend to live in crowded, makeshift refugee camps, which lack sufficient food, safe water, and adequate sanitation. As such, refugee camps become breeding grounds for infectious diseases, malnutrition, and additional violence from unresolved disputes and the presence of small arms.

Disproportionate numbers of women, children, and the elderly are among civilians left behind in wars. Specifically, women and children are the ones most likely to suffer significant excess deaths from such preventable problems as severe malnutrition from food shortages, maternal mortality, epidemics of otherwise vaccine-preventable diseases such as measles, and unexploded ordnance (Ghobarah et al. 2004). Civilian casualties from weapons left behind is a powerful example of how activities of daily life can turn deadly long after battles have ended, due to the negligence of warring parties. For example, according to the United Nations, 2016 saw a steep jump in the number of Afghan children killed or maimed by explosive remnants left by multiple parties to the conflict, during activities such as playing outdoors or attending a wedding (UNAMA 2017, 17).

For both men and women, war decreases life expectancy, creates disabilities, and the "weathering" effects of stress which itself can compromise health through the immune systems and higher rates of mental illnesses such as depression and posttraumatic stress disorder (PTSD) (Geronimus 1996; de Jong et al. 2000). Children who survive wars may represent a future generation living daily with illnesses and injuries that are its direct and indirect results.

Mental Health Costs

At the turn of the new millennium, a report by the World Health Organization (WHO 2001) showed that between one-third and one-half of all persons affected by violent conflicts experience mental distress. PTSD is the most frequent diagnosis. According to the report, PTSD arises "after a stressful event of an exceptionally threatening or catastrophic nature and is characterized by intrusive memories, avoidance of circumstances associated with the stressor, sleep disturbances, irritability and anger, lack of concentration and excessive vigilance" (WHO 2001, 43).

Although many individuals who live through wars may not receive a PTSD diagnosis, it is generally recognized that refugees exhibit particularly high rates of depression, PTSD, and other psychiatric illnesses in comparison to other civilian counterparts in war zones, particularly if they experienced torture (Hamblen and Schnurr 2003). More broadly, wars may cause anxiety and depressive disorders in both the combatant and civilian populations. Rates of acute psychosis and schizophrenia also increase during and in the immediate aftermath of war (WHO 2001). Entire communities under threat of drone attack in Pakistan, for example, experience a physically and emotionally corrosive quotidian terror (Tahir 2013).

Wars frequently lead to self-destructive behaviors and interpersonal violence. Alcohol and substance abuse increase during wartime, perhaps as mechanisms for coping with physical pain or anxiety and other emotional distress, as Anila Daulatzai shows in her chapter on heroin use in Afghanistan. Because of the increased prevalence of weapons, homicide and suicide rates rise within countries during wartime, tending to peak in the first year after a war begins (Ghobarah et al. 2004). As the chapter in this volume by anthropologist Kenneth MacLeish shows, both deployed and non-deployed US service members have experienced a heightened risk of suicide since the United States went to war in Iraq and Afghanistan, due to the stresses of repeated deployments, family conflicts, repeated moves, and physical and emotional wear. Suicide and homicide are intensified by the widespread availability of small arms, including their circulation in refugee camps. Although young men tend to be both the perpetrators and the victims of homicide and suicide, homicide is also a consequence for girls and younger women. Indeed, the chief victims of homicide during wartime are women and younger men (Ghobarah et al. 2004, 879–80).

Social science and public health research conducted in a variety of war-afflicted contexts, including Afghanistan, Algeria, Chad, Lebanon, Sri Lanka, and the West Bank, show that many mental health problems, including pervasive feelings of distress, come not just from armed conflict but also from the "daily stressors" that accompany it, such as "poverty, social marginalization, isolation, inadequate housing, and changes in family structure and functioning" (Miller and Rasmussen 2010, 8).

Furthermore, as Tol et al. (2010) explain, despite the high incidence of mental health problems among those who experience war, the infrastructure and accompanying policy measures needed to treat mental health problems are usually lacking, especially in the low- and middle-income countries where wars typically take place. For example, in Nepal, Tol et al. show how mental health problems stem from contextual factors such as reduced access to basic needs due to conflict, as much as from conflict itself. The pervasive medical focus on the experience of PTSD during and after wartime is far too narrow. As anthropologists Jean Scandlyn and Sarah Hautzinger point out in their ethnographic portrait of a Colorado military community in this volume, "PTSD alone fails to capture the many effects of war on families and communities that cannot be explained by mental illness alone or at all."

Demographic Costs

Because of wartime disruptions in the life trajectories of young men and women, wars have significant demographic consequences. Individuals left behind by their partners end up in extremely vulnerable situations of poverty, economic insecurity, and physical risk. As parents are killed or die of preventable maternal mortality, the number of orphans and female- and child-headed households increases. Additionally, forced or voluntary emigration of significant segments of the population leads to depopulation (Grove and Zwi 2006). These demographic shifts in a postwar society may take decades to resolve, significantly altering the fabric and the social safety nets within a given postwar society. Daulatzai's chapter on Afghan war widows provides an example of how armed conflict leaves women alone and necessitates the formation of new alliances among them that confound NGO policies and popular images of helpless war widows in need of aid. One woman uses heroin in order to numb the pain of the loss of her son in a bomb blast and, later, her husband to a heroin overdose. Another woman uses food rations from the NGO where she is a beneficiary in order to feed an impoverished war widow who now uses heroin as a mode of endurance. In the absence of alternative means to cope, substance use makes sense in this context.

In war, women suffer injuries, reproductive problems, mental health problems, and gender violence, including rape. Tools of warfare include the use of mass rape. Refugee women, removed from social networks that might protect them, are often raped inside and outside of refugee camps, including sometimes by the intergovernmental forces charged with protecting their safety. Medical anthropologist Linda Whiteford (2009) discusses the widespread rape of women in refugee camps during and following the civil wars in Africa and shows how humanitarian aid workers delivering food witnessed this violence against women but felt powerless to do anything to prevent the violence or mitigate its consequences.

Scholars also document the link between armed conflict and intimate partner violence. Men who have suffered from political violence are more likely to be perpetrators of intimate partner violence (Gupta et al. 2009). Annan and Brier (2010) studied women abducted by the Lord's Resistance Army (LRA) in Uganda and showed how these women experienced a great deal of violence after leaving the LRA, including partner violence, because of factors such as poverty that perpetuate conflict. Moreover, psychological factors associated with having suffered rape during their abduction affected these women's future relationships. Children who are enrolled as participants in war, as well as children conceived through war rape, may suffer significant stigma. For example, a study of child soldiers in Sierra Leone showed that post-conflict experiences of discrimination led to increased depression, anxiety, and hostility (Betancourt et al. 2010; see also Theidon 2015).

Women who are raped during periods of war may suffer postwar deaths from cervical cancer and HIV/AIDS, the two conditions that top the list of war-induced health effects for women (Ghobarah et al. 2004). In countries affected by civil war, HIV/AIDS tops the list of war-induced infectious diseases, affecting both genders, especially in the most productive age groups, with devastating impact (ibid.). War-related movements of both refugees and soldiers are heavily implicated in the spread of HIV/AIDS, especially in war-torn parts of sub-Saharan Africa. Women who are infected by HIV/AIDS during wartime may also infect their infants (ibid.).

Women suffer from a host of maternal ills. This includes obstetric emergencies in the absence of adequate wartime healthcare and emergency transport to hospitals. As a result, maternal mortality is high during wartime, amounting to almost one year of healthy life lost per one hundred women in the major child-bearing age group (Ghobarah et al. 2004). The chapter in this book by anthropologist and midwife Kylea Laina Liese shows how the threat of armed violence, lack of access to obstetric care, and women's seclusion in their homes serve to exacerbate already high maternal mortality rates. Recent attempts to train community midwives are encouraging, but they do not go far enough to lessen the risk for women in a climate of social isolation and looming violence.

Social and Infrastructural Costs

War exacts a toll on the social structures that make everyday life predictable and livable, including healthcare systems. As several highly publicized cases in which the United States bombed hospitals in Afghanistan demonstrate, wars entail the random destruction and deliberate military targeting of clinics, hospitals, and laboratories, as well as destruction of the physical infrastructure (e.g., water treatment, electrical systems, transportation infrastructure) necessary to keep health facilities running (Donaldson et al. 2010; Craig, Ryan, and Gibbons-Neff 2015; Medicins sans Frontieres 2015). Wartime destruction of supporting infrastructure impacts the distribution of potable water, food, medicine, relief supplies, and ambulances to healthcare facilities and to refugee camps where populations may be in dire need. Medical anthropologist Mac Skelton's ethnographic chapter about Iraqi cancer patients who must travel to Beirut to access adequate care shows how the quest for life-saving treatment has come to entail separation from family members, economic disenfranchisement, and social dislocation—particularly for those wounded Iraqis whose treatment the government will not fund.

Political priorities during and after war shape peoples' access to healthcare, sometimes regardless of who is most in need of life-sustaining treatment. In this volume, Ghassan Soleiman Abu-Sittah, a plastic and reconstructive surgeon at American University of Beirut Medical Center (AUBMC), uses his in-depth experience with the war wounded from Iraq to show how war wounds are far from simple physical problems to solve but rather do or do not come to light and care through a complicated politics. The Iraqi government pays for healthcare for some wounded Iraqis, including by funding their medical travel abroad, while refusing to do so for others. Who is funded for what kind of care depends vastly on the value that politicians assign to certain war wounds at any given time. As Abu-Sittah tells us, since the takeover of Mosul by ISIS, all patients referred by the Iraqi Ministry of Health (IMOH) to AUBMC's reconstructive surgery services have been members of the Iraqi Army, whereas in the past, the Ministry sent large numbers of Iraqi civilians. Thus, the changing political regime in wartime Iraq has had a tremendous impact on the "war wound itself," including who gets properly referred and treated for injuries that are disabling and life-altering.

Beyond the damage to healthcare's infrastructure, war exacts a great toll on its personnel (Burnham et al. 2012). Military forces often deliberately target doctors and other medical staff, killing and kidnapping them, in order to weaken the opposition. Healthcare providers must make critical decisions about whether to stay and serve during wartime, or to flee with other exiles and refugees. In this volume, as physician Layth Mula-Hussain points out in his public health analysis of increasing cancer rates in Iraq, the epidemic of untreated cancer in the country has been exacerbated by the flight of many of Iraq's medical doctors, including oncologists.

Healthcare systems that have been depleted by war can take years to restore to prewar levels. For example, in Iraq, war combined with the 1990s' UN sanctions to cut off valuable medical supplies such as chemotherapy drugs, and the flight of medical professionals has been compounded by the depletion of healthcare infrastructure over decades. According to Mula-Hussain, between 50 percent and 80 percent of cancers among Iraqis are diagnosed at very late stages of the disease. These patients have few options for state-of-the-art oncological treatment or even palliative care. Mula-Hussain urges action at the highest levels of the Iraqi government to rebuild cancer research and oncology and to prevent needless death and suffering.

Deaths among working-age people, war-related disability, and the flight of people from all walks of life have dramatic impacts on the economic growth of a nation, as well as the basic subsistence of its citizens. Increasing impoverishment and food insecurity during wartime may lead to petty theft and other crimes of poverty (e.g., illegal sex work), as men and women struggle to feed themselves and their families. In general, social safety nets are weakened and even lost during wartime, with family members having to support each other in the absence of government-provided social services (Joseph 2004). As noted by Rylko-Bauer and Singer (2011), war can shred the cultural fabric of a society, including a people's material cultural heritage, identity (particularly sharpening ethnic boundaries which can sometimes be exploited in stoking future conflicts), and set of values that emerged in association with their previous economic and social order, as well as individual livelihoods and life trajectories.

Education comes under attack during war. For millions of children, attending school becomes dangerous, unpredictable, or impossible. Governments may redirect spending from school systems. Teachers and pupils are often unable to reach schools safely due to the real possibility of getting caught in crossfire, raped by parties to the conflict, or specifically targeted for violence to terrorize other students, teachers, and civilians more generally (Global Coalition to Protect Education from Attack 2018). Various parties to conflict use schools as bases, barracks, and strategic points, convert them into makeshift IDP shelters, and destroy them by targeted or indirect fire (ibid.). A May 2018 report by a coalition of eight human rights and humanitarian organizations covering more than forty countries found that targeted and indiscriminate attacks on schools, universities, teachers, and students have grown more widespread over the past five years (2013–2018), compared to prior years covered by the coalition (ibid.).

In the aftermath of war, public health spending may be significantly compromised. Wars typically have a severe short-term (approximately five-year) negative impact on economic growth, reducing financial resources that private sector employers and citizens can devote to health spending. Economic factors both influence the risk of war and affect healthcare spending during and after wartime, as policymakers invest in military buildup with the stated purpose of security and military readiness but divert resources and funding away from environmental protection and restoration, and the development of healthcare systems (Ghoborah et al. 2004).

As discussed above, war zones themselves are not the only places where healthcare systems suffer. Societies that wage wars also sustain the burden of caring for soldiers who return with war wounds. In the United States, an under-resourced, overburdened military healthcare system has been unable to care adequately for returning Iraq and Afghanistan veterans and their many kinds of injuries. They rely heavily on (mostly female) spouses and family members to care for soldiers and veterans. Medical anthropologist Zoë Wool's chapter in this volume turns a critical eye to military healthcare policies that place daily caretaking burdens on (usually male) soldiers' (usually female) partners. She notes how those policies presume the heterosexual family with a female spouse and a male soldier as the basis for care. As in some war zones themselves, moreover, women and families not only assume a large caretaking burden but face an increased risk of falling victim to interpersonal violence from an injured but abusive partner.

Environmental Costs

War, by its destructive nature, also devastates ecosystems, making postwar environmental repair a major challenge. It pollutes air, water, and soil. Environmental toxicity from a variety of chemical weapons (e.g., mustard gas, Agent Orange/dioxin, napalm, depleted uranium) is now recognized as a major potential consequence of conflict (Closmann 2009; Johnston 2007, 2011; Smith 2017). Some of these agents are used in war as defoliants, destroying the vegetation and, along with it, food-producing orchards and energy-providing firewood sources. In addition, war's weapons, such as phosphorus bombs, may pollute the air and leave environmental residues in areas of heavy shelling and bombardment. These toxins also often produce a permanent state of dread of illness: what Johnston (2007, 2) calls "radiogenic communities" are people living with "half-lives"—lives "profoundly affected and altered by a hazardous, invisible threat, where the fear of nuclear contamination and the personal health and intergenerational effects from exposure color all aspects of social, cultural, economic and psychological well-being." That is, they are not only affected by the physical ill health of contaminant exposure or the need to care for kin so affected, but by the daily fear of continued exposure effects, and the stigmatization and humiliation of their victimhood.

Increasingly, reports are beginning to surface about the links between wartime use of chemical agents and negative human health outcomes, including cancer, birth defects, and sterility among war veterans (Gammeltoft 2014; Inhorn 2012; Kilshaw 2008; Manduca, Naim, and Signoriello 2014; Miller 2013). "Scorched-earth" actions undertaken in war, along with radioactive contamination from weapons production and use, may introduce genetic damage into populations (Inhorn 2018). In addition to these threats of environmental toxicity, land mines have been used heavily in some wars, leading to increased death and disability (including limb amputations), primarily among the civilian population (Inhorn and Kobeissi 2006).

The threat of environmental toxicity from weapons is often coupled with the threat of environmental toxicity from waste. Improper waste disposal during war places civilian populations at increased risk of infectious diseases, including those associated with increased pests in the environment (e.g., rodents, flies, and mosquitoes). The modern military bases constructed and used to make war can be among the most polluting entities on earth, with jet fuel and solvents often seeping or spilling into local aquifers, drinking water, and soil. Wartime chaos and the opportunism it allows has sometimes involved dumping of toxic waste from other countries in the war zone, as has also been reported during the Lebanese civil war, when Italian and German companies paid off militia forces to take contaminated waste (Hamdan 2002). Chemicals introduced into the environment during wartime have polluted the air, leached into groundwater aquifers used for drinking water, and polluted the soil used for food crops.

War preparation in the form of massive base-building has had these effects as well and introduced invasive species, destroyed coral reefs and other sea and food resources to devastating effect, and introduced tons of military contaminants to soil and water, as on the island of Guam, for example, the site of major US bases used in long-distance warfare since World War II (Marler and Moore 2011).

Few societies have sufficient resources for environmental cleanup and remediation to deal with the environmental consequences of war (Inhorn and Kobeissi 2006). People often must live with the risk and loss of productive land associated with unexploded ordnance (Henig 2012; Schwenkel 2013), as in the Mariana Islands, where World War II and Cold War toxins and unexploded ordnance have been endemic.

Medical Anthropology: About and Against War

Years into the wars in Afghanistan and Iraq, Marcia Inhorn (2008, 421) asked her fellow American and other medical anthropologists, "Why is there so little on the medical anthropology of [these] war[s]? What is the cause of our inertia?" She was concerned with a lack of anthropological attention to issues in the ongoing war in Iraq and in other parts of the Middle East.

A decade on, a new generation of medical anthropologists has risen to this challenge. Beginning their research careers in the early years of the US-led wars in Iraq and Afghanistan, several young scholars, including some whose work is included in this volume, began focusing on US soldiers and their wounded bodies and psyches (e.g., Finley et al. 2010; Finley 2011; MacLeish 2012; Messinger 2009; Wool 2015; Wool and Messinger 2012). For instance, Zoë Wool (2015) explored how severely injured soldiers rebuild their lives back in the United States, and how their ordinary daily struggles contrast with common narratives of the heroic wounded veteran. Kenneth MacLeish (2012) analyzed the bodily and affective vulnerabilities that military institutions exploit and create in soldiers at Fort Hood, Texas, while Erin P. Finley (2011) examined how veterans diagnosed with PTSD struggle to reconnect with families and mental health services, with some veterans recovering while others do not. These medical anthropology scholars have contributed rich studies on the postwar lives and health impacts of war on US soldiers, lending ethnographic nuance to a field that has been dominated by medicine, public health, and psychiatry, and heavily focused on PTSD (Hoge et al. 2007).

They provide an important response to what anthropologists Arthur Kleinman and Robert Desjarlais (1995, 176) first described as the "medicalization of violence," when medical professionals paint trauma as a universal category of human existence, rooted in individual rather than social dynamics. For instance, Kleinman and Desjarlais critique the aforementioned category of PTSD, which medicalizes the mental health problems resulting from war. When governments and military institutions rely upon and send human beings to engage in acts of war that are otherwise illegitimate and immoral, they treat the resulting problem as one of psychological maladjustment requiring health institutions' intervention. Moreover, the medicalization of violence also violates sufferers' experience of trauma, as medical phrasings often distort the lived experiences of those who suffer from what has been enacted during war (Kleinman 2007). Is a condition like PTSD a disease, or is it simply a normal human reaction to the violence of war, as both observed and perpetrated?

Kleinman and Desjarlais' insights provide a framework for the way medical anthropologists and other analysts have for some time approached violence and mental health. These scholars have sought to politicize casualties born of armed conflict, as the product of public policies and the decisions of political and economic elites. For example, Catherine Panter-Brick (2010) introduced her edited collection on war and health by noting that "determinants of ill-health . . . are patently avoidable, unnecessary, and unfair, necessitating political will and concerted action to meet the human rights objectives of equitable access to health" (1). Medical anthropologist Duncan Pedersen (2002) also highlights the important intersection of health consequences and human rights violations during contemporary wars, wars that are increasingly being fought within states and that target civilians.

As other medical anthropologists have shown, war often exacerbates the negative health consequences of structural violence in impoverished communities and countries, thereby creating new forms of everyday violence. One example of the links between political conflict and structural violence is Ivy Pike and colleagues' (2010) study of the health consequences of low-intensity intercommunity conflict in Kenya. Many of Africa's conflict areas are in pastoralist communities, and ongoing violent conflict there is dominated by small arms like AK47s. In these "small wars," violence has become increasingly routine. Pike and her colleagues argue that bodily, emotional, psychological, and social experiences of this violence are inseparable. They list the direct consequences of violent raids on health: increased fatalities, injuries, and grief/trauma. They also list indirect consequences, including loss of livestock, which leads to distress over loss of identities centered on cattle, impoverishment and hunger, as well as displacements leading to reduced access to resources such as food, water, health clinics, and social networks. Pike and colleagues' work provides an important reminder of how armed violence deepens preexisting inequalities and creates new material, political, and social problems, beyond combat casualties.

Likewise, Catherine Panter-Brick and Mark Eggerman (2012) find that the war-related trauma suffered by Afghan children was not confined to experiences of combat and war-related physical violence, but often to the everyday violence that accompanied it. For example, the domestic violence suffered by children within their families during wartime was a key factor in mental health problems. Panter-Brick and Eggerman demonstrate, as has Theidon (2012) in Peru, that when we focus only on the suffering of war, the remarkable resilience of surviving war can be hidden from view.

In another powerful example of how armed conflict deepens structural violence, Nicole Berry (2012) examines the impact of postwar *violencia* on indigenous women's abilities to access safe obstetric care. In *Unsafe Motherhood: Mayan Maternal Mortality and Subjectivity in Post-War Guatemala*, Berry shows that indigenous communities suffered the most during the long-term Guatemalan civil war, and still suffer in the aftermath, including from pervasive violent crimes and profiling committed against them. Indeed, Mayan women's reluctance to seek healthcare in Guatemala's cities, sometimes during obstetric emergencies, is part of the legacy of their violent treatment by authorities, including medical personnel.

Yet just as war exacerbates structural violence, the reverse may be true; addressing structural violence can help inoculate against war. As Kristian Heggenhougen (2009) argues in his ethnography of Mayan community health workers (CHWs), "a fight against structural violence is also a fight for a safer society" (190). Working amidst political conflict in 1970s Guatemala, CHWs carried the seeds of broader political change (see also Smith-Nonini 2010). They were therefore targeted by a government who viewed them as disturbing the status quo.

Adding perspective to fine-grained ethnographies of war and its impact on local communities are analyses of the role played by the global circulation of people and goods (including weapons) during war. Carolyn Nordstrom (2009) focuses on the health consequences of war for children in some of her work on war and shadow economies in Africa. She tells the story of children orphaned by the Angolan civil war, who are living on the streets. She describes how girls must sell themselves to buy food and medicine, how the children live with the constant threat of violence and exploitation from various groups of adults, and how they treat themselves when they have physical problems by buying medicine from smugglers of pharmaceutical drugs. Nordstrom notes how the horrific health-related hardships these children face are related not just to the political situation in Angola, but to global economic patterns of inequality, such as the exploitations of the pharmaceutical industry.

Nordstrom's work, and that of others, such as Jessaca Leinaweaver's analysis of the international circulation of war-orphaned Peruvian children (2008) and Paul Farmer's (2009) work on the "social life" of land mines in post-genocide Rwanda, point to the need for a global critique of the production of violence. As Farmer explains in telling the story of a Rwandan boy seriously injured by a land mine, basic services like healthcare and education are human rights, and governments and the international aid community should honor them as such. Daniel Hoffman's (2017) observations on the US military's role in global health interventions also demonstrates the importance of understanding how the blurring of the identities of war-maker and healer have resulted in dangerous new forms of transnational militarism, particularly via healthcare crises.

Together, this literature on armed violence and health paints a textured picture of war as encompassing multiple kinds of violence: not only armed violence among state and non-state actors, but also, interpersonal violence and structural violence as well. In his work on post-apartheid South Africa, Didier Fassin (2009, 115) urges anthropologists "to try to recognize violence in the places where it is no longer recognized for what it is" (116). Fassin's observation is relevant to war itself, when governments such as the United States' fail to create "body counts" of direct war mortality in places like Iraq and Afghanistan (Inhorn 2018), or when they fail to acknowledge or document war-induced disease or healthcare infrastructure losses due to war violence. That "national security"-legitimated secrecy is itself a further violence of war that hides the known health effects of war, their scale, and the profits being made from waging war and ignoring its consequences (Nader and Gusterson 2007).

What Is to Be Done?

This varied medical anthropological literature on war and health points to several ways scholars and practitioners might work to alleviate health problems and shape healthcare policy. First, as highlighted by Rylko-Bauer and Singer (2011), healthcare workers can strive to mitigate the direct consequences of war, and also serve to alleviate forms of structural violence that war deepens and exacerbates, by promoting conflict resolution, reconciliation, and peace-building (231). The work of Patricia Omidian (2009), who lived and worked in Afghanistan from 1998 to 2008 doing research for various NGOs, is an example of such a holistic approach to health. So is that of physician-anthropologist Paul Farmer (2004) and his organization Partners in Health who have striven to address poverty, limited access to food sources, and displacement in the war-affected countries where they have worked.

Second, a growing medical anthropology of war and health suggests the fruitfulness of promoting indigenous organizing to create healthcare systems. For example, Sandy Smith-Nonini's (2010) ethnographic account, *Healing the Body Politic: El Salvador's Popular Struggle for Health Rights from Civil War to Neoliberal Peace*, shows how the El Salvador civil war (1980–1992) unexpectedly created the conditions for a new popular healthcare system. With the aid of a liberation force, international NGOs, and the Catholic Church, organizers in the Chalatenango region developed a system in which local health promoters delivered primary care and health education. By the end of the war, one hundred promoters delivered healthcare to 11,000 people, with measured effects in reducing the incidence of basic diseases like diarrhea and increasing vaccine rates.

Third, we can contest the notion that war's victims assume the burden of proof that they have suffered health effects. As Nader and Gusterson (2007) argue, secrecy norms that help prepare for and wage wars must be discarded and instead we must assert the necessity of democratic approaches to death and illness prevention through war prevention.

Fourth, the medical anthropology of war and health suggests the value of culturally sensitive healthcare programs that prioritize local needs and local conceptions of health and healing. The work of Omidian (2009), just referenced, provides one poignant example. Omidian developed a culturally sensitive training program to address trauma and the psychosocial needs of Afghan women, who were struggling with war-related distress and everyday forms of violence.

"Do No Harm"

Of course, once wars occur, there exists a fine line between doing good and doing harm in a context of war zone medicine, particularly when so much of health-related reconstruction aid is administered by nations whose goals are primarily strategic rather than humanitarian or developmental, and by corporations with profit-distorted practices (Lutz and Desai 2015; Guarasci 2017). What happens to healthcare systems postconflict, when countries at war, including Iraq and Afghanistan, have become so dependent on humanitarian assistance driven mainly by such donor interests?

One major issue is the question of sustainability of temporary healthcare aid provided by foreign governments who withdraw after a war's end. For example, Sharon Abramowitz (2015) examines Medicines Sans Frontier's (MSF) withdrawal from Liberia after the end of that country's civil war in 2003. Along with a host of other NGOs, MSF ostensibly worked with Liberia's healthcare sector, but in reality, they provided all the bureaucratic, technical, financial, and logistical support that allowed it to function. After the withdrawal of these NGOs, the local healthcare system could not function because it had no electricity, drugs, supplies, and lab testing capacity.

Further, when humanitarianism substitutes for a failure of political rights, it can have the effect of excluding people from the political body and limiting what it means to be human (Ticktin 2006; see also Fassin 2007). Stuart Gordon (2015), a former member of the British Armed Forces in Iraq, examines the conflicted role of military doctors in Afghanistan. Military doctors are combatants in the fight against insurgents (sometimes firing guns), but they also treat allied soldiers and Afghan combatants. Wounded British or American soldiers are transferred to hospitals abroad, whereas wounded Afghan soldiers are transferred to local hospitals that are not as well equipped as even rudimentary military field stations and where they have fewer chances of survival. Gordon also documents how military medicine is regarded as a threat to civilian medical NGOs operating in Afghanistan. Gordon's ethnography is particularly relevant in highlighting the role of militaries in providing care as well as inflicting violence.

Third, healthcare systems are often viewed by combatants as tools for control. Health workers and infrastructure are targeted by combatants in many conflicts globally (Rylko-Bauer and Singer 2011, 231). Patricia Omidian and Catherine Panter-Brick (2015) describe the ongoing danger experienced by Pakistani healthcare workers, who are targeted by Islamic militants with kidnapping and killing. This has serious consequences, not just for these people and their families, but for the instance when, in 2012, Pakistan suspended its polio eradication campaign after nine polio fieldworkers were killed. Unlike expatriates, local aid workers have few safety nets, and travel with little protection. Women health workers in particular are endangered.

Finally, in what Rylko-Bauer and Singer (2011, 234) call the "dark side" of healthcare in war, scholars have documented the involvement of medical professionals in war—for example, in the cooptation of medicine in the Third Reich, or in colonial sanitation campaigns (Rylko-Bauer 2009; Sidel 1996). Most recently, in the US war in Iraq, medical professionals have been involved in the torture of detainees. Scholars also have critiqued the use of medical outreach campaigns as ways of winning hearts and minds in counterinsurgency campaigns (Bloche 2016).

Questioning War

Given the many "dark sides" of war, it is important to reiterate the call for anthropologists to question the legitimacy of particular wars like that in Iraq or Afghanistan and the very legitimacy of war itself (Inhorn 2008; Lutz and Millar 2012).

War budgets direct funds toward military institutions and away from health and social needs (Holden 2017; Lutz 2002). In Iraq and Afghanistan, the United States has spent (or has been obligated to spend, in the case of future veterans' healthcare and disability payments) approximately $5.9 trillion on the wars (Crawford 2018a)—money that could have been spent to counter growing inequality in the United States; to repair roads, bridges, and schools; to invest in clean energy development; and to hire more workers in human service sectors such as education and health (Garrett-Peltier 2017). As war diverts revenue into military spending, it also restructures budgets for decades after it is "over" as money must be spent to deal with a population's war injuries that are disabling for a lifetime, or with destroyed infrastructure. All of this expense is encountered at the same time that government revenues are diminished as a result of economic disruptions and losses.

Simultaneously, wars destroy the built and natural environments in which people live. Armed conflict creates environmental danger zones, such as landmine fields, and degrades environments, with significant impact on human health through the pollution of potable water sources, the creation of literally tons of toxic waste by advanced militaries, including spilled jet fuels and solvents and radioactive armaments used and abandoned in the environment (Inhorn 2018; Smith 2017). Wars also, as already discussed, have indirect effects on health through the destruction of housing, healthcare facilities, and social and physical infrastructure. This includes the running of sewage through once-clean streets after the bombing of treatment plants (Al-Mohammad 2007).

In this context of diminished financial resources and environmental destruction, wars cause trauma and injury to civilians, including children, who are particularly vulnerable and who suffer chronic mental health and physical health problems because of their experiences (Singer and Hodge 2010). There are many undocumented casualties—people who die through paramilitary action, torture rooms, civilian concentration camps, and the like (ibid.). As an example of the kinds of uncounted casualties that Singer and Hodge stress, as many as one million Vietnamese people today suffer from cancers, genetic disorders, and other disabilities as a result of exposure to Agent Orange during the Vietnam War (Gammeltoft 2014).

Indeed, the institution of war damages and destroys human bodies as a central goal and most horrific consequence. That this even needs to be pointed out requires explanation, as Elaine Scarry (1987) notes. How can people—from government officials to the general public—so often speak of war first and foremost as a contest between nations or generals, or ultimately "about" a struggle for territory, resources, or ideological purity? How can the bodily harm be seen simply as a side consequence of the pursuit of loftier political goals, or baser economic ones?

The reasons are many, but most centrally, it is because wars would be more difficult to prosecute if, from the outset, the thousands or even millions of dead or injured bodies were emphasized. In the era of modern warfare, a government's population cannot be continually reminded of war's "central fact" (dead and injured bodies), because of the contemporary assumption, particularly in the United States and Europe, that their states and their wars have been benevolent in intent and deeply committed to the protection of civilians.

To examine war and its effects on human health, we need to first navigate around this tendency to ignore the bodies damaged by war, and the push by governments for publics to instead focus on the love between military "brothers," on the beautiful spectacle of war pyrotechnics, on the religious or secular sentiments of nationalist pride at the protecting army, or the fear and anger at the threat of harm from others.

An Opening Example: Health Costs of War in Iraq

Over the past decade, the Iraq war in particular has inspired work by both medical anthropologists and public health scholars, who have documented the destruction of Iraq's healthcare system and examined the health consequences of war there in painful detail (Dewachi 2011; Dewachi et al. 2014; Dewachi 2017; Inhorn 2018).

Scott Harding and Kathryn Libal (2010) provide important historical context. During the 1960s and 1970s Baathist period in Iraq, Iraq invested heavily in its health sector. By the 1980s, it was outperforming many European countries in its health indicators, despite the heavy tolls of the Iraq-Iran war (1980–1988). However, in the First Gulf War of 1990–91, US bombing campaigns destroyed extensive parts of Iraq's infrastructure, and the ensuing UN sanctions period (1990–2003) took its toll on the country's medical infrastructure and public health. By the time of the 2003 US invasion, the public health system in Iraq was already functioning very poorly.

However, since the 2003 US invasion, Iraq has been in the midst of a true public health crisis. Despite a formal mission of improving Iraqis' well-being, the US military presence has only worsened public health by further impoverishing Iraqis and underinvesting in infrastructure. Harding and Libal (2010) document some of the damaging health consequences of the 2003 invasion. Health indicators in Iraq show high rates of mortality among both combatants and civilians, rising child and infant mortality, and the reliance of one-third of Iraqis on emergency healthcare services in a country once known for its excellent primary healthcare sector. Degraded water and sanitation systems have led to disease outbreaks; food insecurity and malnutrition are now rampant; and most local healthcare facilities have very poor operating conditions. Violent conflict has led to high rates of displacement—more than 2 million Iraqis in neighboring countries, more than 3 million internally displaced, and as many as 11 million in need of humanitarian assistance (Edwards 2016).

Furthermore, the 2003 US invasion triggered massive internal destabilization and increasing sectarianism. Iraqis fear everyday violence from armed sectarian groups, criminals, militias, and various military forces, and therefore have difficulty accessing the few public services that exist. Security risks delay service delivery, such as ambulance transport, and prevent Iraqis' access to hospitals and clinics. Harding and Libal (2010) also note that the militant targeting of Iraqi medical professionals has led to a brain drain in the healthcare sector, with few left to train new healthcare professionals.

Notably, healthcare in Iraq is not just an unintended casualty of the US-led invasion. US and allied forces have actively undermined health infrastructure as part of their military strategy in the country: Both American and British military forces have sometimes attacked key public health infrastructure, such as hospitals, ambulances, bridges, and homes (Hills and Wasfi 2010). US forces have also radically downsized the Iraqi public sector and attempted to privatize public services, which has led to further corruption and inefficiencies, and further reduced Iraqis' access to healthcare.

Because of these direct and indirect assaults on the Iraqi healthcare system, including severely diminished access to food and water, children have been greatly affected by war. They have not been immunized, many are underweight and malnourished, and at the height of the war only 40 percent had access to safe drinking water. "In 2005, one in eight Iraqi children died of disease or violence in the first five years of life," as noted by Hills and Wasfi (2010, 133). By 2007, 4 million Iraqis were deemed "food insecure" (133).

Furthermore, environmental pollution is now rampant in Iraq. Communicable diseases have spread because of sewage contamination of water sources (Hills and Wasfi 2010; Al-Mohammed 2007). In addition, US armaments used in the First Gulf War and the chemical and conventional weapons used since 2003 have created toxic pollution, including radioactive contamination, which is believed to have carcinogenic and genotoxic health effects (Hills and Wasfi 2010).

Mental illness, suffering, and trauma have accompanied many aspects of the 2003 US-led war in Iraq. Iraq is now a country of widespread insecurity, not only from the ongoing military violence, but from rampant assassinations and kidnappings among Iraqis in all sectors of society (Hills and Wasfi 2010). Those Iraqis who have fled the violence and insecurity are uprooted, facing the difficulties of internal displacement and refugee resettlement, and the inability to return to their homes.

Health Consequences of the Wars in Afghanistan and Pakistan: An Introduction

The US military and its NATO allies have maintained an on-the-ground presence in Afghanistan since 2001. The forces fighting that alliance work across the border with Pakistan and to ensure that government's cooperation, the United States has spent billions of dollars to help fund and supply the Pakistani military in its fight against Islamist insurgents, not least of all through drone strikes in the border regions with Afghanistan which have killed tens of thousands of insurgents as well as civilians (Haqqani and Curtis 2017; Afzal 2013; Costs of War Project 2016). Simultaneously, national and international aid organizations and UN agencies have established a network of hospitals, clinics, and awareness-raising campaigns to provide information and healthcare to ill and injured civilians throughout Afghanistan and in the border regions between Afghanistan and Pakistan, in many respects filling a public health void carved by decades of war and underinvestment in human services in these regions.

In Afghanistan and in the Pakistani border regions most affected by the wars, the humanitarian and public health situation remains dire. In

2016, Amnesty International reported that the number of people internally displaced by the ongoing conflict had doubled to 1.2 million in three years, with most lacking access to basic healthcare services, adequate food, and potable water, and most women giving birth in unsanitary conditions without any skilled help (Amnesty International 2016). Many internally displaced persons in Afghanistan face exposure to extreme and life-threatening weather conditions (ibid.). Key public health indicators are poor, with one in three Afghan children malnourished (Costs of War Project 2016).

Pakistan is a major receiving country for Afghan refugees, many of whom face constant insecurity and threats of deportation from the Pakistani government, severe malnourishment, and lack of access to healthcare and adequate housing in Pakistani refugee camps (Human Rights Watch 2017; Borgen Project 2014). In addition, a combination of ongoing armed conflict, natural disasters such as flash floods and earthquakes, and lack of government investment in primary healthcare in the region have contributed to poor public health indicators among Pakistani civilians living in these border regions. For example, as of 2015, Pakistan had an under-5 mortality rate of 78.8 children per 1,000 live births, and a maternal mortality rate of 178 women per 100,000 live births (World Health Organization 2016). As Coburn and Closser's chapter in this volume shows, most people in the border regions of Federally Administered Tribal Areas (FATA) and Khyber Pakhtunkhwa (KPK) lack access to basic primary and preventative healthcare.

Given this context of ongoing insecurity and poverty, the four chapters in this book on the health effects of the wars in Afghanistan and Pakistan further help to answer the questions: Have international humanitarian interventions, in partnership with local government and personnel, developed a healthcare system that will last after troops and aid workers eventually leave, and in a context of ongoing insecurity? What are the unintended consequences of so many different military and public health actors alighting in this region with their own agendas?

Both military and international public health campaigns have accomplished some of their goals. Drone strikes have killed high-profile leaders with connections to the Taliban, and polio vaccination campaigns have inoculated many children against polio in one of the last regions in the world where cases of the disease are still found. Yet military and public health campaigns have also sown widespread distrust among Pakistanis and Afghans who see them as connected. Closser and Coburn's chapter on drone strikes, mentioned above, is a case in point: Many Pakistani families in border regions view visits from internationally funded vaccination workers as another foreign intrusion into their lives, a possible provocation of violence from local insurgents, and a diversion of resources from primary healthcare and psychological assistance.

Understandably, many Afghans and Pakistanis retreat to kin and social networks to meet their health needs. For example, Liese discusses how in remote Afghan villages, young women rely on their mothers-in-law during childbirth rather than skilled midwives or hospital staff, because of the dangers of venturing outside of the home after decades of state- and militia-sponsored violence. Home births also serve to strengthen familial relationships that enable women to survive and that provide meaning.

These pieces and others in this volume, such as Daulatzai's chapter on Afghan widows, show that people benefit most from available care only when providers respect their understandings of sickness and healing. Sickness in this region cannot be understood only in terms such as maternal deaths, polio cases, and drug addiction (as in the case of Daulatzai's chapter), but as rooted in the chronic insecurity of war, lack of access to primary care, and governments' and donors' failure to prioritize investments in such care and the infrastructure, such as roads, that people need to access it in the first place.

Likewise, healing demands more than just vaccines, substance abuse treatment, and safe access to hospitals and midwives, among other things. In the cases elaborated in this book, preconditions for resilience include freedom from social stigma, inclusion in families and friendships, the sense of meaning that comes from the ability to help people who are more vulnerable, and access to culturally relevant psychosocial support, among other examples.

Conclusion

Far into their second decade, these wars in Iraq and Afghanistan have become "permanent." Afghanistan has become the site of the longest war in modern US history, followed by the war in Iraq. The United States had also joined wars in Libya, Syria, and Yemen, and in 2017 posted troops to eighty countries in its global counterterror war (Savell et al. 2019). Their health effects are not only historical facts but are ongoing.

The contributors to this volume have begun the work of understanding how two twenty-first-century wars have affected human health for Afghans and Iraqis alike, as well as the US military personnel who were commanded to fight there. The chapters in this volume move chronologically beginning with Afghanistan, which the United States invaded in 2001; then moving to Iraq, which the United States invaded in 2003; and then to Pakistan, where the United States began its campaign of drone warfare in 2004; and ending in the United States, whose soldiers continue to return from these ongoing conflicts. The number of chapters devoted to each national health context should not be interpreted to suggest anything like an equality of scale of human suffering in each of those locations but rather the availability of currently existing ethnographic research into those contexts.

Many of the long-term health consequences of war are still not well understood, and may take generations to uncover, much less ameliorate. Yet clearly, the current wars in Afghanistan and Iraq, and the lingering effects of serial[1] and co-occurring wars (such as the "War on Drugs" in Afghanistan) in both of those countries, continue to haunt and disrupt the lives of millions of people, and inscribe continuing effects on individuals' bodies. War has been a cause of profound human suffering in Afghanistan, Iraq, and Pakistan, but has also adversely affected the American war veterans and US-paid war contractors who went home from Iraq and Afghanistan with bodily and psychic injuries. We hope ultimately to communicate how the decision to go to war—and to stay at war—is catastrophic to human health and ecosystems. In this light, wars cannot, in any meaningful sense, be won.

This volume forms part of the project of recognizing the violence of war, so that scholars and practitioners can use their work to help work against it. It covers a wide scope of direct and indirect health casualties of the ongoing wars in Afghanistan, Iraq, and Pakistan. Its authors show how the wars exact suffering among those who fight them as well as their families; on the battlefield and far beyond it; in the war zones, where healthcare has been decimated by serial conflict, and in the United States, where healthcare infrastructure is highly developed.

So, while our case studies focus on the post–9/11 wars, this introduction demonstrates that there is an important global story to be told about how widely and deeply war affects individuals, families, and communities. For example, the American spouse who leaves her job to care for a chronically injured veteran may have experiences in common with the Afghan widow who learned to be a breadwinner for her family, following her husband's war-related suicide. The Iraqi family who must live apart so that an uncle with cancer can receive adequate care in Lebanon may be somewhat like Angolan families forcibly separated by decades of conflict, coping with life's hardships apart. The Afghan woman who struggles to access basic prenatal care in a war-ravaged, deeply conservative society might share aspects of her struggle with indigenous Guatemalan women who fear accessing state health services following years of government counterinsurgency operations. The US veteran who, in 2050, will still be struggling with the limits of the amputations from his long past injuries in an IED attack in Afghanistan will be living a life parallel to that of an Afghan policeman, although that Afghan will be even more challenged and impoverished by decades of unemployment as a result of his disabling war injuries as well as his country's devastated condition. In painting a picture of the post–9/11 wars and their health consequences, we hope to prompt readers to think further and more globally about the health consequences of all wars, and to take real steps to alleviate those consequences or, more pressingly, prevent new ones.

NOTE

1 See Anila Daulatzai's chapter in this volume for a more detailed discussion of the term "serial war."

REFERENCES

Abramowitz, Sharon. 2015. "What Happens When MSF Leaves? Humanitarian Departure and Medical Sovereignty in Postconflict Liberia." In *Medical Humanitarianism: Ethnographies of Practice*, edited by Sharon Abramowitz and Catherine Panter-Brick, 137–154. Philadelphia: University of Pennsylvania Press.

Afzal, Madiha. 2013. "Drone Strikes and Anti-Americanism in Pakistan." *Brookings*, February 7. Retrieved from www.brookings.edu.

Al-Mohammad, Hayder. 2007. "Ordure and Disorder: The Case of Basra and the Anthropology of Excrement." *Anthropology of the Middle East* 2 (2): 1–23.

Amnesty International. 2016. "'My Children Will Die This Winter': Afghanistan's Broken Promise to the Displaced." Retrieved from www.amnesty.org.

Annan, Jeannie, and Moriah Brier. 2010. "The Risk of Return: Intimate Partner Violence in Northern Uganda's Armed Conflict." *Social Science and Medicine* 70 (1): 152–59.

Barker, Holly. 2004. *Bravo for the Marshallese: Regaining Control in a Post-Nuclear, Post-Colonial World*. Belmont, CA: Wadsworth/Thomson Learning.

Berry, Nicole. 2012. *Unsafe Motherhood: Mayan Maternal Mortality and Subjectivity in Post-War Guatemala*. New York: Berghahn.

Betancourt, Theresa S., Jessica Agnew-Blais, Stephen E. Gilman, David R. Williams, and B. Heidi Ellis. 2010. "Past Horrors, Present Struggles: The Role of Stigma in the Association between War Experiences and Psychosocial Adjustment among Former Child Soldiers in Sierra Leone." *Social Science and Medicine* 70 (1): 17–26.

Bloche, M. Gregg. 2016. "When Doctors First Do Harm." *New York Times*, November 22.

Borgen Project. 2014. "Health Issues Grow for Afghan Refugees." Retrieved from borgenproject.org.

Burnham, Gilbert, Sana Malik, Ammar S. Dhari Al-Shibli, Ali Rasheed Mahjoub, Alya'a Qays Baqer, Zainab Qays Baqer, Faraj Al Qaraghuli, and Shannon Doocy. 2012. "Understanding the Impact of Conflict on Health Services in Iraq: Information from 401 Iraqi Refugee Doctors in Jordan." *International Journal of Health Planning and Management* 27: e51–e64.

Closmann, Charles E. 2009. *War and the Environment: Military Destruction in the Modern Age*. College Station: Texas A&M University Press.

Costs of War Project. 2016. Brown University. http://watson.brown.edu/costsofwar.

———. 2017. Brown University. Retrieved from http://watson.brown.edu/costsofwar.

———. 2018. Brown University. Retrieved from http://watson.brown.edu/costsofwar.

Craig, Tim, Missy Ryan, and Thomas Gibbons-Neff. 2015. "By Evening, a Hospital. by Morning, a War Zone." *Washington Post*, October 10. Retrieved from www.washingtonpost.com.

Crawford, Neta. 2016. "Update on the Human Costs of War for Afghanistan and Pakistan, 2001 to mid-2016." Retrieved from http://watson.brown.edu/costsofwar.

———. 2018a. "United States Budgetary Costs of the Post-9/11 Wars Through FY2019: $5.9 Trillion Spent and Obligated." Retrieved from http://watson.brown.edu/costsofwar.

———. 2018b. "The Ripple Effects of Attacking Infrastructure in War: Afghanistan and Iraq." Paper presented to the Annual Meeting of the International Studies Association, April.

———. 2018c. "Human Cost of the Post–9/11 Wars: Lethality and the Need for Transparency." Costs of War Project. Retrieved from http://watson.brown.edu/costsofwar.

Daponte, Beth Osborne. 1993. "A Case Study in Estimating Casualties from War and Its Aftermath: The 1991 Persian Gulf War." *Physicians for Social Responsibility Quarterly* 3: 57–66. Retrieved from www.ippnw.org.

de Jong, J. P., W. F. Scholte, M.W.J. Koeter, and A.A.M. Hart. 2000. "The Prevalence of Mental Health Problems in Rwandan and Burundese Refugee Camps." *Acta Psychiatrica Scandinavica* 102: 171–77.

Dewachi, Omar. 2011. "Insecurity, Displacement and Public Health Impacts of the American Invasion of Iraq." Retrieved from http://watson.brown.edu/costsofwar.

———. 2017. *Ungovernable Life: Mandatory Medicine and Statecraft in Iraq*. Stanford, CA: Stanford University Press.

Dewachi, Omar, Mac Skelton, Vinh-Kim Nguyen, Fouad M. Fouad, Ghassan Abu Sitta, Zeina Maasri, and Rita Giacaman. 2014. "Changing Therapeutic Geographies of the Iraqi and Syrian Wars." *The Lancet* 383 (9915): 449–57.

Donaldson, Ross I., Yuen Wai Hung, Patrick Shanovich, Tariq Hasoon, and Gerald Evans. 2010. "Injury Burden During an Insurgency: The Untold Trauma of Infrastructure Breakdown in Baghdad, Iraq." *Journal of Trauma—Injury, Infection and Critical Care* 69: 1379–85.

Edwards, Adrian. 2016. "Global Forced Displacement Hits Record High." *United Nations High Commissioner for Refugees*, June 20. Retrieved from www.unhcr.org.

Farmer, Paul. 2004. *Pathologies of Power: Health, Human Rights, and the New War on the Poor*. Oakland: University of California Press.

———. 2009. "'Landmine Boy' and the Tomorrow of Violence." In *Global Health in Times of Violence*, edited by Barbara Rylko-Bauer, Linda Whiteford, and Paul Farmer, 41–62. Santa Fe, NM: School for Advanced Research Press.

Fassin, Didier. 2007. "Humanitarianism as a Politics of Life." *Public Culture* 19 (3): 499–520.

———. 2009. "A Violence of History: Accounting for AIDS in Post-apartheid South Africa." In *Global Health in Times of Violence*, edited by Barbara Rylko-Bauer, Linda Whiteford, and Paul Farmer, 113–36. Santa Fe, NM: School for Advanced Research Press.

Finley, Erin P. 2011. *Fields of Combat: Understanding PTSD among Veterans of Iraq and Afghanistan*. New York: ILR Press.

Finley, Erin P., Monty Baker, Mary Jo Pugh, and Alan Peterson. 2010. "Patterns and Perceptions of Intimate Partner Violence Committed by Returning Veterans with Post-Traumatic Stress Disorder." *Journal of Family Violence* 25 (8): 737–43.

Gammeltoft, Tine. 2014. *Haunting Images: A Cultural Account of Selective Reproduction in Vietnam*. Berkeley: University of California Press.

Garrett-Peltier, Heidi. 2017. "Job Opportunity Cost of War." Retrieved from http://watson.brown.edu/costsofwar.

Geneva Declaration Secretariat. 2008. *Global Burden of Armed Violence*. Cambridge: Cambridge University Press.

———. 2015. *Global Burden of Armed Violence*. Cambridge: Cambridge University Press.

Geronimus, Arline. 1996. "Black/White Differences in the Relationship of Maternal Age to Birthweight: A Population-Based Test of the Weathering Hypothesis." *Social Science and Medicine* 42: 589–97.

Ghobarah, Hazem Adam, Paul Huth, and Bruce Russett. 2004. "The Post-War Public Health Effects of Civil Conflict." *Social Science and Medicine* 59 (4): 869–84.

Global Coalition to Protect Education from Attack (GCPEA). 2018. Education Under Attack, 2018. New York: Global Coalition to Protect Education from Attack.

Gordon, Stuart. 2015. "The British Military Medical Services and Contested Humanitarianism." In *Medical Humanitarianism: Ethnographies of Practice*, edited by Sharon Abramowitz and Catherine Panter-Brick, 176–90. Philadelphia: University of Pennsylvania Press.

Grove, Natalie J., and Anthony B. Zwi. 2006. "Our Health and Theirs: Forced Migration, Othering, and Public Health." *Social Science and Medicine* 62: 1931–42.

Guarasci, Bridget. 2017. "Environmental Rehabilitation and Global Profiteering in Wartime Iraq." April 23. *Costs of War*. Retrieved from www.watson.brown.edu/costsofwar.org.

Gupta, Jhumka, Dolores Acevedo-Garcia, David Hemenway, Michele R. Decker, Anita Raj, and Jay G. Silverman. 2009. "Premigration Exposure to Political Violence and Perpetration of Intimate Partner Violence Among Immigrant Men in Boston." *American Journal of Public Health* 99 (3): 462–69.

Hamblen, Jessica, and Paula Schnurr. 2003. "Mental Health Aspects of Prolonged Combat Stress in Civilians: A National Center for PTSD Fact Sheet." *PTSD: National Center for PTSD*. Retrieved from www.ptsd.va.gov.

Hamdan, Fouad. 2002. "The Ecological Crisis in Lebanon." In *Lebanon's Second Republic: Prospects for the Twenty-first Century*, edited by Kail C. Ellis, 175–87. Gainesville: University Press of Florida.

Haqqani, H., and L. Curtis. 2017. "A New U.S. Approach to Pakistan: Enforcing Aid Conditions without Cutting Ties." *Hudson Institute*. Retrieved from www.hudson.org.

Harding, Scott, and Kathryn Libal. 2010. "War and the Public Health Disaster in Iraq." In *The War Machine and Global Health: A Critical Medical Anthropological Examination of the Human Costs of Armed Conflict and the International Violence Industry*, edited by Merrill Singer and G. Derrick Hodge, 59–88. Lanham, MD: Altamira Press.

Heggenhougen, H. Kristian. 2009. "Planting 'Seeds of Health' in the Fields of Structural Violence: The Life and Death of Francisco Curruchiche." In *Global Health in Times of Violence*, edited by Barbara Rylko-Bauer, Linda Whiteford, and Paul Farmer, 181–200. Santa Fe, NM: School for Advanced Research Press.

Henig, David. 2012. "Iron in the Soil: Living with Military Waste in Bosnia-Herzegovina." *Anthropology Today* 28 (1): 21–23.

Hills, Elaine A., and Dahlia S. Wasfi. 2010. "The Causes and Human Costs of Targeting Iraq." In *The War Machine and Global Health: A Critical Medical Anthropological Examination of the Human Costs of Armed Conflict and the International Violence Industry*, edited by Merrill Singer and G. Derrick Hodge, 119–56. Lanham, MD: Altamira Press.

Hoffman, Daniel J. 2017. "Military Humanitarianism and Africa's Troubling 'Forces for Good.'" *Insights*, May 16. Retrieved from items.ssrc.org.

Hoge, Charles W., Artin Terhakopian, Carl A. Castro, Stephen C. Messer, and Charles C. Engel. 2007. "Association of Posttraumatic Stress Disorder with Somatic Symptoms, Health Care Visits, and Absenteeism among Iraq War Veterans." *American Journal of Psychiatry* 164 (1): 150–53.

Holden, Paul. 2017. *Seven Myths that Sustain the Global Arms Trade*. London: Zed Books.

Human Rights Watch. 2017. "Pakistan Coercion, U.N. Complicity: The Mass Forced Return of Afghan Refugees." February 13. Retrieved from www.hrw.org.

Inhorn, Marcia C. 2008. "Medical Anthropology against War." *Medical Anthropology Quarterly* 22 (4): 416–24.

———. 2012. *The New Arab Man: Emergent Masculinities, Technologies, and Islam in the Middle East*. Princeton, NJ: Princeton University Press.

———. 2018. *America's Arab Refugees: Vulnerability and Health on the Margins*. Stanford, CA: Stanford University Press.

Inhorn, Marcia C., and Loulou Kobeissi. 2006. "The Public Health Costs of War in Iraq: Lessons from Post-war Lebanon." *Journal of Social Affairs* 23: 13–47.

Johnston, Barbara Rose, ed. 2007. *Half-Lives and Half-Truths: Confronting the Radioactive Legacies of the Cold War*. Santa Fe, NM: School for Advanced Research Press.

———. 2011. *Life and Death Matters: Human Rights, Environment, and Social Justice*. 2nd ed. New York: Routledge.

Joseph, Suad. 2004. "Conceiving Family Relationships in Post-War Lebanon." *Journal of Comparative Family Studies* 35: 271–93.

Kilshaw, Susie. 2008. *Impotent Warriors: Perspectives on Gulf War Syndrome, Vulnerability and Masculinity*. Oxford and New York: Berghahn Books.

Kleinman, Arthur. 2007. *What Really Matters: Living a Moral Life Amidst Uncertainty and Danger*. Oxford: Oxford University Press.

Kleinman, Arthur, and Robert Desjarlais. 1995. "Violence, Culture, and the Politics of Trauma." In *Writing at the Margin: Discourse between Anthropology and Medicine*, edited by Arthur Kleinman, 173–92. Berkeley: University of California Press.

Lafta R., S. Al-Shatari, M. Cherewick, L. Galway, C. Mock, A. Hagopian, et al. 2015. "Injuries, Death, and Disability Associated with 11 Years of Conflict in Baghdad, Iraq: A Randomized Household Cluster Survey." *PLoS ONE* 10(8): e0131834. doi.org/10.1371/journal.pone.0131834.

Leinaweaver, Jessaca. 2008. *The Circulation of Children: Kinship, Adoption, and Morality in Andean Peru*. Durham, NC: Duke University Press.

Lutz, Catherine. 2002. "Making War at Home in the United States: Militarization and the Current Crisis." *American Anthropologist* 104 (3): 723–35.

Lutz, Catherine, and Sujaya Desai. 2015. "US Reconstruction Aid for Afghanistan: The Dollars and Sense." *Costs of War Project*. Retrieved from http://watson.brown.edu/costsofwar.

Lutz, Catherine, and Kathleen Millar. 2012. "War." In *A Companion to Moral Anthropology*, edited by Didier Fassin, 482–99. New York: Blackwell.

MacLeish, Kenneth T. 2012. "Armor and Anesthesia: Exposure, Feeling, and the Soldier's Body." *Medical Anthropology Quarterly* 26 (1): 49–68.

Manduca, Paola, Awny Naim, and Simona Signoriello. 2014. "Specific Association of Teratogen and Toxicant Metals in Hair of Newborns with Congenital Birth Defects or Developmentally Premature Birth in a Cohort of Couples with Documented Parental Exposure to Military Attacks: Observational Study at Al Shifa Hospital, Gaza, Palestine." *International Journal of Environmental Research and Public Health* 11 (5): 5208–23. Retrieved from www.mdpi.com.

Marler, Thomas E., and Aubrey Moore. 2011. "Military Threats to Terrestrial Resources Not Restricted to Wartime: A Case Study from Guam." *Journal of Environmental Science and Engineering* 5 (9): 1198–1214.

Medicins sans Frontieres. 2015. *Initial MSF Internal Review: Attack on Kunduz Trauma Centre, Afghanistan*. Retrieved from www.doctorswithoutborders.org.

Messinger, Seth D. 2009. "Incorporating the Prosthetic: Traumatic, Limb-loss, Rehabilitation and Refigured Military Bodies." *Disability and Rehabilitation* 25 (31): 2130–34.

Miller, Kenneth E., and Andrew Rasmussen. 2010. "War Exposure, Daily Stressors, and Mental Health in Conflict and Post-Conflict Settings: Bridging the Divide between Trauma-Focused and Psychosocial Frameworks." *Social Science and Medicine* 70 (1): 7–16.

Miller, Robert. 2013. "Respiratory Disorders Following Service in Iraq." Retrieved from http://watson.brown.edu/costsofwar.

Nader, Laura, and Hugh Gusterson. 2007. "Nuclear Legacies: Arrogance, Secrecy, Ignorance, Lies, Silence, Suffering, Action." In *Half-Lives and Half-Truths: Confronting the Radioactive Legacies of the Cold War*, edited by Barbara Rose Johnston. Santa Fe, NM: School for Advanced Research Press.

Nordstrom, Carolyn. 2009. "Fault Lines." In *Global Health in Times of Violence*, edited by Barbara Rylko-Bauer, Linda Whiteford, and Paul Farmer, 63–88. Santa Fe, NM: School for Advanced Research Press.

Omidian, Patricia A. 2009. "Living and Working in a War Zone: An Applied Anthropologist in Afghanistan." *Practicing Anthropology* 31 (2): 4–11.

Omidian, Patricia, and Catherine Panter-Brick. 2015. "Dignity Under Extreme Duress: The Moral and Emotional Landscape of Local Humanitarian Workers in the Afghan-Pakistan Border Areas." In *Medical Humanitarianism: Ethnographies of Practice*, edited by Sharon Abramowitz and Catherine Panter-Brick, 23–40. Philadelphia: University of Pennsylvania Press.

Ostrach, Bayla, and Merrill Singer. 2013. "Syndemics of War: Malnutrition-Infectious Disease Interactions and the Unintended Health Consequences of Intentional War Policies." *Annals of Anthropological Practice* 36 (2): 257–73.

Panter-Brick, Catherine. 2010. "Conflict, Violence, and Health: Setting a New Interdisciplinary Agenda." *Social Science and Medicine* 70 (1): 1–6.

Panter-Brick, Catherine, and Mark Eggerman. 2012. "Understanding Culture, Resilience, and Mental Health: The Production of Hope." In *The Social Ecology of Resilience: A Handbook of Theory and Practice*, edited by Michael Unger, 369–86. New York: Springer.

Pedersen, Duncan. 2002. "Political Violence, Ethnic Conflict, and Contemporary Wars: Broad Implications for Health and Social Well-Being." *Social Science and Medicine* 55: 175–90.

Pike, Ivy L., Bilinda Straight, Matthias Oesterle, Charles Hilton, and Adamson Lanyasunya. 2010. "Documenting the Health Consequences of Endemic Warfare in Three Pastoralist Communities of Northern Kenya: A Conceptual Framework." *Social Science and Medicine* 70 (1): 45–52.

Rylko-Bauer, Barbara. 2009. "Medicine in the Political Economy of Brutality." In *Global Health in Times of Violence*, edited by Barbara Rylko-Bauer, Linda Whiteford, and Paul Farmer, 201–22. Santa Fe, NM: School for Advanced Research Press.

Rylko-Bauer, Barbara, and Merrill Singer. 2011. "Political Violence, War, and Medical Anthropology." In *A Companion to Medical Anthropology*, edited by Merrill Singer and Pamela I. Erikson, 219–50. West Sussex: Blackwell.

Savell, Stephanie and 5W Infographics. 2019. "Where We Fight." *Smithsonian Magazine*, February: 58–59.

Scarry, Elaine. 1987. *The Body in Pain: The Making and Unmaking of the World*. Oxford: Oxford University Press.

Schwenkel, Christine. 2013. "War Debris in Postwar Society: Managing Risk and Uncertainty in the DMZ." In *Interactions with a Violent Past: Reading Post-Conflict Landscapes in Cambodia, Laos, and Vietnam*, edited by Vatthana Pholsena and Oliver Tappe, 135–56. Singapore: NUS Press.

Sidel, Victor W. 1996. "The Social Responsibilities of Health Professionals: Lessons from Their Role in Nazi Germany." *Journal of the American Medical Association* 276 (20): 1679–81.

Singer, Merrill, and G. Derrick Hodge, eds. 2010. "Introduction: The Myriad Impacts of the War Machine on Global Health." In *The War Machine and Global Health: A Critical Medical Anthropological Examination of the Human Costs of Armed Conflict and the International Violence Industry*, edited by Merrill Singer and G. Derrick Hodge, 1–30. Lanham, MD: Altamira Press.

Smith, Gar, ed. 2017. *The War and Environment Reader*. Charlottesville, VA: Just World Books.

Smith-Nonini, Sandy. 2010. *Healing the Body Politic: El Salvador's Popular Struggle for Health Rights from Civil War to Neoliberal Peace*. New Brunswick, NJ: Rutgers University Press.

Tahir, Madiha. 2013. *Wounds of Waziristan*. Film. Retrieved from woundsofwaziristan.com.

Theidon, Kimberly. 2012. *Intimate Enemies: Violence and Reconciliation in Peru*. Philadelphia: University of Pennsylvania Press.

———. 2015. "Hidden in Plain Sight: Children Born of Wartime Sexual Violence." *Current Anthropology* 56 (12): S191–200.

Ticktin, Miriam. 2006. "Where Ethics and Politics Meet: The Violence of Humanitarianism in France." *American Ethnologist* 33 (1): 33–49.

Tol, Wietse A., Brandon A. Kohrt, Mark J. D. Jordans, Suraj B. Thapa, Judith Pettigrew, Nawaraj Upadhaya, and Joop T.V.M. de Jong. 2010. "Political Violence and Mental

Health: A Multi-Disciplinary Review of the Literature on Nepal." *Social Science and Medicine* 70 (1): 35–44.

United Nations Assistance Mission in Afghanistan (UNAMA). 2017. *Afghanistan Annual Report on Protection of Civilians in Armed Conflict: 2016*. February. Retrieved from unama.unmissions.org.

Whiteford, Linda. 2009. "Failure to Protect, Failure to Provide: Refugee Reproductive Rights." In *Global Health in Times of Violence*, edited by Barbara Rylko-Bauer, Linda Whiteford, and Paul Farmer, 89–112. Santa Fe, NM: School for Advanced Research Press.

Wool, Zoë. 2015. *After War: The Weight of Life at Walter Reed*. Durham, NC: Duke University Press.

Wool, Zoë, and Seth D. Messinger. 2012. "Labors of Love: The Transformation of Care in the Non-Medical Attendant Program at Walter Reed Army Medical Center." *Medical Anthropology Quarterly* 26 (1): 26–48.

World Health Organization. 2001. *The World Health Report 2001—Mental Health: New Understanding, New Hope*. Geneva: World Health Organization.

———. 2016. "Pakistan Key Indicators." Retrieved from apps.who.int.

PART I

Afghanistan and Pakistan

1

Childbirth in the Context of Conflict in Afghanistan

KYLEA LAINA LIESE

Decades of social upheaval and protracted violence have taken tolls on both the public sector and private life in Afghanistan. Women, in particular, have endured vulnerabilities and assaults to their personhoods, livelihoods, and bodies. In 2002, Afghanistan's maternal mortality ratio (MMR) was among the highest in the world at 1,600 per 100,000 live births (Bartlett et al. 2005), with nearly 92 percent of all births taking place without access to a skilled birth attendant (Newbrander et al. 2014). Since 2002, the Afghan government, several nongovernmental organizations (NGOs), and the US government have committed tremendous resources to developing a national healthcare delivery system. The resulting BPHS (Basic Package Health Services) dramatically expanded the reach of maternal healthcare, and midwifery care, in particular. Between 2003 and 2009, the number of Afghans living within a two-hour walk of basic healthcare increased from 9 percent to 85 percent (Ministry of Public Health 2010).[1] The number of midwives increased from 467 to more than 4,600 (UNFPA 2014). Afghanistan's maternal mortality ratio is still among the highest in the world, but vastly lower than it was at the start of the war: 400 maternal deaths per 100,000 live births (WHO et al. 2015).

The reduction in maternal mortality between 2003 and 2009 would not appear nearly as impressive if Afghan women's health had not been in such a deplorable state prior to 2002. This chapter explores the macro- and micro-aggressions by which war and social instability have made Afghan women among the most vulnerable in the world. Although access to lifesaving obstetric care may be essential to treat complications arising in pregnancy and birth, the maternal mortality ratio in Afghanistan in 2002 indicated the problem went well beyond poverty and infrastructure to the long-lasting and far-reaching impact of violence.

Researchers have observed that armed conflicts and postwar conditions amplify the health detriments of poverty and increase risk for maternal mortality through a variety of mechanisms, including reduced access to obstetric care and contraception, increased risk of infectious disease, and higher levels of malnutrition. One study found that the mean adjusted MMR in sub-Saharan African countries subject to recent armed conflict (since 1990) was 1,000/100,000 births, while countries without recent conflict had a mean MMR of 690/100,000 (O'Hare and Southall 2007). What social and historical conditions allowed for such pathology in physiologic childbirth? How do war and violence directly and indirectly jeopardize women's reproductive health?

Major political changes in Afghanistan over the last 30 years made Afghan women's lives and reproduction largely invisible. At the national level, public policies restricting women's roles in society limited infrastructure and access to reproductive health services. The Taliban issued edicts that shut down medical and nursing schools for girls and women, while also forbidding female doctors from working and female patients from seeing male physicians. Afghan women were also required to wear the burqa and be accompanied by a male relative when outside the home or risk public beatings for disobedience. The consequences of these policies reverberate deeply into the private sphere, reinforcing power dynamics within the family unit. In order to "protect" their daughters from external threats that included violence and kidnapping, families sought earlier marriages than had been the norm (Liese 2009). Marriage conveyed protection for young girls, though their new families also controlled their autonomy and livelihoods. In the absence of trained midwives and doctors, authoritative knowledge of pregnancy and childbirth fell upon family members who lacked healthcare skills but were responsible for helping a woman give birth in the safety of the home. The social context of wartime added meaning to childbirth, protecting and strengthening kin ties during a time when external threats were both unpredictable and pervasive. However, this seclusion also made women more vulnerable socially and physically.

In her notable essay, "Do Muslim Women Really Need Saving? Anthropological Reflections on Cultural Relativism and Its Others," Abu-Lughod cautions us against conflating the causes of Afghan women's "continuing malnutrition, poverty, and ill health, and their more recent exclusion under the Taliban from employment, schooling, and the joys of wearing nail polish" (Abu-Lughod 2002, 784). She rightfully acknowledges that throughout South Asia, Africa, and the Middle East, colonialism utilized the notion of liberating women from repressive cultural practices in order to justify itself. The Soviet Union, which occupied Afghanistan from 1979 to 1989, propagated Muslim women throughout Central Asia as a "surrogate proletariat" to be liberated from the shackles of Islam by communist ideology (Northrop 2003). Indeed, it was not the obligation of the burqa or seclusion imposed by the Taliban in the name of religion that caused women in Afghanistan to die during childbirth. Afghan women, particularly those in rural areas, suffered from health disparities common to poverty long before the Taliban took control of the country. The war between the Soviet Union and Afghanistan killed between 900,000 and 1.25 million Afghans (Khalidi 1991). Guerrilla warfare in rural areas by the US-propped mujahedeen and retaliatory air strikes by the USSR leveled villages and decimated farms. By the mid-1990s, the Taliban-installed restrictions, exacerbated by the social history of violence and instability, had additional harmful effects on the health and social lives of Afghan women who had long been vulnerable due to malnutrition, poverty, and ill health.

The dominant public health paradigm views maternal mortality as the result of discrete physiologic causes and individual risk factors, such as maternal age, parity (number of prior pregnancies), education, and socioeconomic status (Maine and Rosenfield 1999). From this perspective, maternal risk is addressed by making obstetric care universally available and accessible to treat obstetric emergencies. Anthropological research on maternal mortality instead focuses on the relationships between the *site-specific* social context of childbirth (Jordan 1997) and public health efforts to reduce maternal risk. Why would people give birth at home when a hospital could save their life? The answers to this question are multifaceted and overlapping. They range from historically rooted structural inequalities (lack of roads, resources, and education and poverty more generally) to sociocultural complexities (discrimination, tradition, values, beliefs). Despite the high rate of maternal mortality in rural postwar Guatemala, Berry (2010) found that women and their families resisted biomedical intervention because it disrupted the social benefits of a home birth as a time to establish and strengthen essential kin networks. This finding was echoed in Hay's (1999) work on maternal mortality in Indonesia, where sociocultural forces contributed to the local perception that the biomedical clinic did not represent the most appropriate care in an obstetric emergency.

This analysis is based on ethnographic data collected between 2006 and 2010 in the Badakhshan Province of northern Afghanistan. I draw on data from hospital records and observations, semi-structured interviews with Afghan women, men, and healthcare workers, a district-wide maternal mortality survey using the sisterhood method, and seventeen months of participant observation in the mountainous regions of Gorno-Badakhshan, Tajikistan, and Badakhshan, Afghanistan. I use these data to argue war and extensive periods of instability create social conditions that increase women's vulnerability during pregnancy and childbirth. They limit access to care directly and indirectly through infrastructure, security, and education. The social context of violence also reinforces insular family dynamics that isolates young women for their own protection, further limiting access to skilled attendance during and following childbirth.

Public Policy, Education, and Healthcare Infrastructure

Changes in healthcare for Afghan women over several decades of civil war reflect larger sociopolitical instability occurring throughout the nation. During the 1970s and 1980s, female physicians, scientists, civil servants, and educators served the Afghan public alongside their male counterparts. With the collapse of the Democratic Republic of Afghanistan in 1992, and subsequent integration of Gulbuddin Hekmatyar as prime minister of the Islamic State of Afghanistan in 1996, the stature and visibility women had gained in the public sector during the communist era quickly eroded. In 1998, the government of Afghanistan issued a decree ordering "householders to blacken their windows, so women would not be visible from the outside" (Rashid 2000). Under the state authority of the Taliban from 1996 to 2001, women were forbidden from working, attending school, or leaving the house without an appropriate male escort. They were instructed in how they should dress, behave, and interact, in order to preserve their honor and that of their families. Judgments about women's movements and propriety were handed out by local thugs who threatened offenders with violent beatings on the street. This state of pervasive instability and extrajudicial violence had both direct and indirect effects on women's ability to receive reproductive healthcare.

The Feyzebod District Hospital is the only hospital in the vast mountainous province of Badakshan. Due to threats of landslides, avalanches, and mudslides, the road to the hospital was only accessible to many parts of Badakhshan a few months of the year. When it was open, the journey from districts near the Tajikistan border could take up to ten days along narrow trails. During the Soviet-Afghan war (1979–1989) and subsequent Afghan civil war (1989–1996), vandals and improvised explosive devices (IEDs) made the road even more perilous.

The hospital suffered a lack of regular personnel and equipment. In order to safely perform a life-saving cesarean section, an obstetrician and anesthesiologist were as vital as medication, surgical equipment, electricity, and running water. But as the civil war stretched from years to decades, medical personnel, supplies, and basic infrastructure dwindled. Because women were forbidden to receive medical care from male doctors, a few female physicians were permitted to practice, but within a climate of fear, violence, and surveillance. One female physician in the northern province of Badakhshan arrived at the Feyzebod District Hospital, where she worked as an obstetrician, wearing an "Arab-style" abaya that covered her entire body except her face, instead of the burqa.[2] She was met at the entrance by a mujahideen who pressed his Kalashnikov against her forehead, telling her he would remove her face if she did not cover it. Threats and harassment like this kept the majority of capable female physicians confined to their homes and away from practicing medicine. Some physicians who had resources chose to leave the country, creating a "brain drain" from which the country has yet to recover.[3] As a result, even if a woman who had permission and an escort to the hospital during an obstetric emergency managed to survive the long journey, she could be sure neither that a provider would be there to treat her, nor that necessary supplies would be available.

By excluding women from attending work and school, the Taliban not only directly prohibited women from access to healthcare, but also stunted the country's ability to meet healthcare needs in the future. For more than five years under the Taliban, female students were prohibited from attending medical or nursing colleges, while male medical students lacked basic educational materials and reported daily harassment and deplorable conditions (Radio Free Europe / Radio Liberty 2006; Rashid 2000).[4] The Taliban's prohibition of girls attending school may have indirectly increased maternal mortality. One study found female secondary school education and trained delivery assistance to be the strongest predictors of national maternal mortality, even when controlling for income per capita (Shiffman 2000). This finding is supported by national survey data collected in 2010–11 by UNICEF and the Afghan government's Central Statistics Organization. The more educated an Afghan woman is, the more likely she is to give birth with a skilled attendant, and therefore more likely to survive childbirth. She is also more likely to delay marriage and pregnancy, further reducing her maternal risk (Oates 2013). In 2006, only 18 percent of Afghan females ages 15 to 24 were literate enough to understand short, simple written sentences on their everyday life (UNESCO Institute for Statistics 2016).[5]

There are likely several mechanisms by which female education protects women's reproductive health. Education increases women's visibility and engagement with public institutions, officials, and bureaucracies, increasing society's accountability toward women. Education empowers individuals and may help women to recognize complications, negotiate assistance, advocate for skilled care, and utilize family planning—all of which decreases maternal risk. One woman in Afghan Badakhshan described the labor of her daughter-in-law: "She had pain in her back and in her stomach. She sat like that for four days. The old woman told her to walk around the room but she was bleeding. We gave her some tea and some opium because it was cold, but she died. The baby did not come out" (Liese 2009). Access to obstetric care necessary to save this woman's life ultimately may have been determined by structural inequalities, including poor road conditions in her district and the unavailability of medical resources within the nearest hospital. Nevertheless, when women are educated, they are more likely to recognize obstetric complications sooner. Earlier recognition of this woman's obstructed labor may have given her time to be transported to a facility. Likewise, education increases the access and availability of skilled providers, minimizing delays and structural barriers to care. Access to skilled providers, such as trained midwives, *within* the community improve chances of surviving an obstetric emergency, but to accomplish this distribution, girls from rural communities must have education opportunities.

Contexts of Violence, Authoritative Knowledge, and Maternal Risk

The impact of violence and war is often represented in quantitative terms: numbers of lives lost, percentage of communities impacted, dollars necessary to rebuild infrastructure. Unrepresented by these data are the ways in which long wars impact community and individual perceptions, actions, and daily practices. Experiences of trauma, fear, and violence persist beyond traditional recovery efforts and shape how actors engage with aspects of everyday life, including health, nutrition, and social relationships. For example, one of the most surprising findings of this research concerns Afghan women's perception of risk in childbirth. Despite having the highest maternal mortality ratio ever recorded (6,507 maternal deaths per 100,000 live births) and a one-in-three risk of dying in childbirth (Bartlett et al. 2005), women interviewed in the Badakhshan province of Afghanistan did not perceive childbirth as extraordinarily dangerous or necessarily life-threatening in comparison with the rest of their lives. In part, this may be an artifact of the gap between epidemiology and lived experience. Although maternal mortality is calculated across the province as the number of deaths per 100,000 live births, in villages of 200 to 300 people, maternal deaths are rare events from the perspective of individual community members. Like other poor, rural, post-conflict communities that suffer comorbidities—such as those resulting from a lack of clean drinking water, food shortages, and insecurity (Berry 2010)—women in Badakhshan were more concerned with day-to-day survival than their less obvious risk of dying in childbirth. Moreover, as Afghans live in large extended patrilineal households, women are surrounded by mothers-in-law, sisters-in-law, and aunts, most of whom have had and survived multiple pregnancies—living proof of maternal survivorship.

When newly married Afghan women move from their natal homes into those of their husbands, the responsibility for their protection is also transferred from their parents to their husbands and in-laws. This responsibility takes priority in times of violence and social upheaval, so much so that it can reduce the age at which girls are married. In Badakhshan, the sparsely populated mountains meant that communities had little warning of when violence would arrive, often in the form of armed groups of men on horseback. Early in the conflict, these groups would be mujahideen fighters, sent to harass and interrogate villagers as to whether they were living according to Shari'a law. Other times, they were bandits posing as Taliban and transporting heroin across Badakhshan and out of Afghanistan's northern border. Unmarried girls were targeted for kidnapping and forced marriage.

Being isolated in the peripheral mountains of Afghanistan, villagers have no effective way to assess the political climate of the central government in real time. This uncertainty meant people in Badakhshan had little sense of how close or far the fight was, exactly who was in charge, or whether the war had ended altogether. When armed men arrived in their villages, they were at their mercy. The effects of these raids on women and their health were twofold. First, it created a climate of fear, mistrust, and auto-surveillance within the community that continued long after the violence stopped. In 2007, while working in a small village in Badakhshan, I stayed with a well-respected family. The mother in the household was one of the only women in the village with any formal education and had been given the title of "Leader of Women." One afternoon, I asked her if she would come with me to a small kiosk only about 20 yards from the house that was owned by her cousin. She explained that we would have to wait till her son or husband returned home. I was surprised that even years after the Taliban left power, she still needed permission and an escort, especially in her small village where she was well known and respected. She explained that during the height of the Taliban, neighbors reported on each other if someone behaved in a way that was not permitted, in order to demonstrate their loyalty and confer protection. Reportable offenses included women leaving the house unaccompanied or dressing immodestly. When Taliban would arrive in the town, the offending party and her family would be severely beaten as punishment.

This efficient system of auto-surveillance persisted, keeping women secluded in their homes and mistrusting of their neighbors, although it had been more than five years since the village had seen violence from outsiders entering their village. Although some assert that the threat of violence from the Taliban ended in 2001, it is impossible for Afghans in peripheral villages to know for certain. As Donna Goldstein (2003) demonstrates in her work on everyday life amidst gang violence in Brazilian favelas, protective mechanisms and practices developed during long waves of violence do not simply disappear during periods of peace. For years, women and men in rural Afghanistan feared unpredictable violent repercussions for disobeying restrictions on women imposed by both the Taliban and mujahideen. Although both groups insisted these restrictions were ordained by Islam, individual men and women continued to follow the rules out of ingrained senses of fear and mistrust. In fact, the most charged symbols of women's invisibility during the wars and after (e.g., the *chodar*, the practice of seclusion, arranged child marriage, female exclusion in education and employment) may be explained as continuing artifacts of violence and isolation.[6] The well-respected mother who cannot walk 20 yards from her home was not concerned that this behavior was immodest or inappropriate, but rather that someone may use those justifications against her if the Taliban or mujahideen returned to their village.

Although seclusion is an artifact of historical violence intended to be protective, the isolation increases the social and physical vulnerability of women and children. Nisso was a small-framed seventeen-year-old with auburn hair who arrived at a local clinic with a crying child in her arms. She explained that her daughter was nearly two years old but very small and not yet walking. She had refused to nurse, and the family had little food. Nisso and her daughter lived with her husband, a man with a white beard who appeared to be in his late fifties or early sixties, who had been widowed without children before marrying Nisso. Her mother-in-law had died before the wedding, Nisso explained, and their home was remote, a full day's walk from the clinic, with no close neighbors. As a result, she spent all of her time alone and inside the mud house. She gave birth unassisted in their home. Afterward, she struggled to care for and nurse the infant, and she was not sure what to feed her child. The midwife in the clinic lifted the child's dress and shook her head as she pointed out the child's limp skin and protruding skeleton. A doctor who was brought in explained the child was severely malnourished and dehydrated. She would die if she was not given IV fluids immediately. If she had open access to a network of women, neighbors, family members, or healthcare workers, Nisso would have better resources during childbirth and information about nursing and infant nutrition. Persistent seclusion makes women nearly invisible over the course of their married lives. Women become dependent on their families for nutrition, information, and healthcare. While most families are deeply invested in supporting their wives and daughters-in-law, this reliance makes women and their children highly vulnerable. The seclusion of women functions as another barrier to the protective factors of education as well as skilled assistance during childbirth.

The second consequence of the uncoordinated attacks on the villages during the civil wars was to reduce the age of marriage. Several women in the village remembered times during and after the Afghan-Soviet war (1979–89) and Afghan civil wars (1989–96) when young girls would be taken as extra wives by armed strangers. By marrying these girls off at younger ages to local men, there was less risk they would be snatched from their parents' homes. As one woman explained, "If people knew that your daughter was very pretty, then a Mujaheed would come to your house on a horse and he would take your daughter from your arms. It is better that she walk to her husband's house when she is still small than be taken away." Since attending school was prohibited, early marriage was even more clearly in the best interest of the child to help ensure their protection. In a focus group of seven women, there was consensus that girls should be married by twelve years old, even though some were married at seven or eight years. Most women described child marriage in the historical context of protecting girls from outside threats, though a few women suggested child marriage was also a custom intended to keep girls out of trouble. Some degree of variation in how women understand the origin of this practice is expected. Significantly, however, the marriage of young girls was never attributed to Islamic practice or interpretation.

Marriage age is an interdependent factor in maternal risk. The earlier a woman is married, the less likely she is to attend school and to have the health and social benefits that formal education confers, but also the sooner she is likely to become pregnant. Women younger than eighteen years old are at higher risk for pregnancy-related complications such as preeclampsia and obstructed labor. Early age at first pregnancy also increases the likelihood of having more children over the course of the reproductive life span. The threat of unpredictable violence that encouraged earlier marriages also served to increase maternal risk. However, with each successful pregnancy, the woman also gains experience and confidence in the processes of labor and birth. If she has managed to deliver healthy children at home without skilled assistance, she may reject the need for her daughter-in-law to deliver in a clinic. Likewise, each time she survives childbirth, the threat that it may kill her appears to diminish. Despite this perception, women's lifetime risk of dying in childbirth in Afghan Badakhshan is one in three (Bartlett et al. 2005).

However, when a school opened in one village in Badakhshan, some families decided to delay their daughters' marriages in favor of completing their education. Delaying marriage in favor of education may have significant impact on overall maternal mortality by increasing the visibility of girls, reducing overall fertility, reducing risky early pregnancies, and making women more capable of recognizing complications. Built with governmental, non-governmental, and donor funds, the school signaled and symbolized a sociopolitical stability that had not been present for decades. For the families who made the choice to send their daughter to school, the benefit of education, once available, outweighed the risk of delayed marriage in current conditions.

Although secondary education increases women's statistical likelihood of having a safer pregnancy and skilled attendance at birth, appropriate providers are still largely inaccessible to most Afghan women. Nevertheless, several distinct systems of knowledge inform Afghan women's decisions related to pregnancy and childbirth. They include biomedicine, traditional Afghan medicine, religious teaching, and personal experience. These systems may complement each other but oftentimes some systems carry more weight than others. Authoritative knowledge in pregnancy and childbirth is not necessarily the knowledge that is "correct" but rather the knowledge that "counts" in a particular situation (Jordan 1997). Authoritative knowledge is the system of knowledge upon which decisions are made and actions are taken, often at the dismissal of other kinds of knowing. In hospitals, authoritative knowledge of whether a cesarean section is necessary often embeds with the physician and biomedicine, perhaps at the expense of the experiential knowledge of relatives in the room. However, what makes authoritative knowledge important is not that it is accurate or necessarily will lead to good outcomes, but that it is accepted and holds status within a particular social group. In the absence of representation of an alternative system of knowledge, such as a midwife or doctor, Afghan mothers-in-law consolidate authoritative knowledge related to pregnancy and childbirth. Their repeated and successful deliveries reinforce their expertise and their authority in asserting that childbirth is a normal life event. In essence, their survival is living proof that childbirth is not that risky and that they can be relied upon to make decisions for the new mother. Furthermore, mothers-in-law already hold authority via their position of power in the household.

In times of violence and instability, the family network is a social safety net vital for protection and survival. Childbirth is a social event whereby the pregnant woman's complete reliance on the authoritative knowledge of her husband and in-laws reinforces these ties. The process of birthing a new family member helps strengthen extended family cohesion, reproducing the family's means to survive during recurrent social instability and violence (Berry 2010).

Childbirth represents a state of liminality, primarily for the mother but also for her child, and her family. As Turner (1969, 94) explains, "Liminal entities are neither here nor there; they are betwixt and between the positions assigned and arrayed by law, custom, convention, and ceremonial." When a woman goes into labor, she is (quite literally) in transition between the changing and codified roles of pregnancy and motherhood. Yet, until the child is born and takes her first breath, the outcome or success of this transition is uncertain. One husband I interviewed observed that a woman in labor is "a woman between life and death." She must pass through this state of liminality within the larger social context of the family and society. When decisions are made during childbirth, the family not only considers the immediate risk to the mother, but the risk of seeking external assistance. The concern generated over persistent bleeding must be weighed against the safety of traveling on the roads, both in terms of road quality issues but also threats of attack.

The authoritative knowledge imbued in the family during pregnancy is powerful, in part, because it extends beyond the childbirth process. The gendered hierarchy of the family where the in-laws are responsible for protecting the daughter-in-law is reinforced during childbirth, as a transitional state where those kin relationships are strengthened. When the threat of violence is external to the household, the household becomes the seat of trust and safety. Relying on each other during birth and trusting the authoritative knowledge extends to the larger social context in which the birth takes place and into which the family will transition.

Conclusion

The wars in Afghanistan destroyed schools, homes, cities, ancient artifacts, roads, and countless lives. The treatment of women became a focal point for international media and scholarship, which linked the gender oppression represented by burqas, seclusion, child marriage, and exclusion from work and school to deplorable health statistics around maternal mortality, malnutrition, and illiteracy. However, the full story of the wars and their aftermath goes beyond popularized images or demographic costs. When the Taliban were removed from power in 2002, health and social indicators improved. Clinics and schools were built and rebuilt, allowing more girls the opportunity for education and healthcare.

The relationships between improved health and well-being indicators and the routing of the Taliban are not so clear-cut. Periods of sustained violence and instability reshape how families and communities relate to each other and the state. Badakhshan did not suffer the consistent violence as provinces in the East and South. But the looming threat of unknown violence created a climate of fear and mistrust that reinforced women's seclusion, reduced marriage age, and consolidated authoritative knowledge within the family unit. These are further examples of the multiple routes by which war creates syndemics (Ostrach and Singer 2013) indirectly and directly damaging human health, causing emotional and social trauma, and destroying physical infrastructure. In order to overcome the threat, families must be convinced the benefits of education and healthcare can outweigh the risk of recurrent violence as communities struggle to live normal lives. For much of rural Afghanistan, the threat of bride kidnappings and armed violence by thugs has changed significantly with the fall of the Taliban and establishment of a centralized government. The number of clinics is growing in peripheral areas, with more opportunities for skilled attendance at birth with community midwives. As schools are built and clinics staffed, Afghanistan has the potential not only to offer treatment for obstetric emergencies but to unravel some of the histories that made women more vulnerable to begin with. Yet, for decades the wars in Afghanistan shaped local perception that the dominant risks facing women were social and external, best managed by the authoritative knowledge of family members who had themselves survived the liminal state of pregnancy. The fear of violence and the structures that were created to protect families do not go away simply because the threat of violence has changed, temporarily. In a country where violence has ebbed and flowed for more than fifty years, people remain wary of changing norms that offer safety and security. The resurgence of violence and Taliban control of certain provinces perhaps validates these concerns. However, recent programs to locally recruit and formally train community midwives establish a culturally acceptable presence of young, female, educated clinicians in rural communities, who are symbolic of both structural and cultural possibilities. That the midwives are recruited and sanctioned by local leaders conveys a social protection to the midwives themselves and families who choose to utilize them. Strengthening their position as part of the community during times of peace may enhance their resilience and ability to protect women should violence return.

NOTES

1 The Special Inspector General for Afghanistan Reconstruction (SIGAR) found inaccuracies in the geospatial coordinates provided by USAID that indicated nearly 80 percent of the new clinics were not located where they had been reported. USAID identified a critical error in their data that led to the inaccurate GPS coordinates and later provided updated coordinates for the clinics. SIGAR also took issue with conditions at 4 of 23 clinics visited which they noted lacked water and electricity. USAID has not publicly responded.

2 The burqa, or chodari, was originally a form of covering used by mostly rural Pashtun women from a region in Southern Afghanistan and was uncommon among women in the North before the war.

3 Another wave of "brain drain" currently threatens Afghanistan as recent gains by the Taliban have propelled a wave of migration to Europe and prompted government-sponsored social media campaigns to dissuade people from leaving the country.

4 Each day the Taliban measured the length of students' beards and turbans, beating the students who were noncompliant. The Taliban also asserted that working

with cadavers was prohibited under Shari'a law. Without anatomy textbooks, students reported digging up graves and stealing bones for their studies. It was not until 2006 that Kabul Medical University graduated (90) female physicians, the first class since 1996 (Radio Free Europe 2006).

5 An assessment of the actual impact of improved female education on maternal health is complicated by endemic corruption in the monitoring and evaluation of governmental and non-governmental programs in Afghanistan. An audit by the Special Inspector General for Afghanistan Reconstruction raises questions regarding whether actual student enrollment is as high as reported by USAID, a primary funding source for education in Afghanistan (SIGAR 2016). Despite this, ethnographic data demonstrate how local schools and community midwives can reduce maternal risk, and international data demonstrate a strong relationship between female education and maternal health (e.g., Lule et al. 2005).

6 Perhaps these fears are no longer warranted. Afghan Badakhshan enjoys relative stability and freedom from the endemic violence that persists in other parts of the country. However, what constitutes a period of stability and peace? If a society has been at war for decades, does five years subjectively constitute the end of violence, or simply a lull (Goldstein 2003)?

REFERENCES

Abu-Lughod, Lila. 2002. "Do Muslim Women Really Need Saving? Anthropological Reflections on Cultural Relativism and Its Others." *American Anthropologist* 104 (3): 783–90.

Bartlett, Linda A., Shairose Mawji, Sara Whitehead, Chadd Crouse, Suraya Dalil, Denisa Ionete, and Peter Salama. 2005. "Where Giving Birth Is a Forecast of Death: Maternal Mortality in Four Districts of Afghanistan, 1999–2002." *The Lancet* 365 (9462): 864–70.

Berry, Nicole S. 2010. *Unsafe Motherhood: Mayan Maternal Mortality and Subjectivity in Post-War Guatemala.* New York: Berghahn Books.

Goldstein, Donna M. 2003. *Laughter Out of Place: Race, Class, Violence, and Sexuality in a Rio Shantytown.* Berkeley: University of California Press.

Hay, M. Cameron. 1999. "Dying Mothers: Maternal Mortality in Rural Indonesia." *Medical Anthropology* 18: 243–79.

Jordan, Briggite. 1997. "Authoritative Knowledge and Its Construction." In *Childbirth and Authoritative Knowledge*, edited by Robbie E. Davis-Floyd and Carolyn Sargent, 55–79. Berkeley: University of California Press.

Khalidi, Noor Ahmand. 1991. "Afghanistan: Demographic Consequences of War, 1978–1987." *Central Asia Survey* 10 (3): 101–26.

Liese, Kylea Laina. 2009. "Motherdeath in Childbirth: Explaining Maternal Mortality on the Roof of the World." PhD diss., Stanford University.

Lule, Elizabeth, Ramana, G.N.V. Ramana, Nandini Ooman, Joanne Epp, Dale Huntington, and James E. Rosen. 2005. *Achieving the Millennium Development Goal of*

Improving Maternal Health: Determinants, Interventions and Challenges. Washington, DC: World Bank Human Development Network.

Maine, Deborah, and Allan Rosenfield. 1999. "The Safe Motherhood Initiative: Why Has It Stalled?" *American Journal of Public Health* 89 (4): 480–82.

Ministry of Public Health, Afghanistan. 2010. *A Basic Package of Health Services for Afghanistan*. Kabul: Ministry of Public Health.

Monitoring and Evaluation Department. 2008. *Afghanistan Health Indicators Fact Sheet—August 2008*. Kabul: Ministry of Public Health.

Newbrander, William, Kayhan Natiq, Shafiqullah Shahim, Najibullah Hamid, and Naomi Brill Skena. 2014. "Barriers to Appropriate Care for Mothers and Infants during the Perinatal Period in Rural Afghanistan: A Qualitative Assessment." *Global Public Health* 9 (S1): S93–S109.

Northrop, Douglas. 2003. *Veiled Empire: Gender and Power in Stalinist Central Asia*. Ithaca, NY: Cornell University Press.

Oates, Lauryn. 2013. *The Education Wager*. Victoria: Canadian Women for Women in Afghanistan.

O'Hare, Bernadette, and David Southall. 2007. "First Do No Harm: The Impact of Recent Armed Conflict on Maternal and Child Health in Sub-Saharan Africa." *Journal of the Royal Society of Medicine* 100 (12): 564–70.

Ostrach, Bayla, and Merrill Singer. 2013. "Syndemics of War: Malnutrition-Infectious Disease Interactions and the Unintended Health Consequences of Intentional War Policies." *Annals of Anthropological Practice* 36 (2): 257–73.

Radio Free Europe / Radio Liberty. 2006. "RFE/RL Afghanistan Report." *Radio Free Europe / Radio Liberty* 5 (14). Retrieved from www.globalsecurity.org.

Rashid, Ahmed. 2000. *Taliban: Islam, Oil and the New Great Game in Central Asia*. New Haven, CT: Yale University Press.

Shiffman, Jeremy. 2000. "Can Poor Countries Surmount High Maternal Mortality?" *Studies in Family Planning* 31 (4): 274–88.

Special Inspector General for Afghan Reconstruction (SIGAR). 2016. "Primary and Secondary Education in Afghanistan: Comprehensive Assessments Needed to Determine the Progress and Effectiveness of Over $759 Million in DOD, State, and USAID Programs." Washington, DC: SIGAR 16-32 Audit Report.

Turner, Victor. 1969. "Liminality and Communitas." In *The Ritual Process: Structure and Anti-Structure*, edited by Victor Turner, 94–113. Chicago: Aldine.

UNESCO Institute for Statistics. 2016. *Youth Literacy Rate, Population 15–24 Years Female (%)*. World Bank Group. Retrieved from data.worldbank.org.

UNFPA. 2014. *State of Afghanistan's Midwifery*. Kabul: UNFPA.

WHO, UNICEF, UNFPA, World Bank Group, and United Nations Population Division. 2015. *Maternal Mortality in 1990–2015: Afghanistan*. Geneva: WHO.

2

Drone Strikes and Vaccination Campaigns

How the War on Terror Helps Sustain Polio in Afghanistan and Pakistan

SVEA CLOSSER AND NOAH COBURN

The images are in striking contrast: The polio vaccination worker going door to door, providing oral vaccination drops to young children, and the smoldering remains of a house, destroyed in the night by a US drone strike. Both of these, however, are products of international interventions in the frontier regions of Afghanistan and Pakistan. Though the ideas and motives behind the two are in some ways worlds apart, planned by very different people in different conference rooms elsewhere, these two programs have become deeply entangled on the ground.

The recent decades of conflict in Afghanistan and Pakistan have had broad impacts on the health of Afghans and Pakistanis. The most obvious are the direct casualties of war, with more than 200,000 killed by violence directly from the war and many more injured (see appendix and Crawford 2018). But these numbers, as shocking as they are, are the tip of the iceberg. War's wider impacts on human lives, from forced displacement to food insecurity to the destruction of health facilities, are far greater than war's direct casualties. These kinds of health effects are often so large and diffuse as to be nearly impossible to enumerate.

Examining the wars' effects on just one disease can allow for a closer approximation and understanding. The border region between Pakistan and Afghanistan is one of the last places on earth where polio continues to infect children, paralyzing their limbs and sometimes killing them. The Global Polio Eradication Initiative—a coalition of the Pakistani and Afghan governments, the World Health Organization (WHO), UNICEF and other international organizations—spends more than $200 million a year in the area, vaccinating large numbers of children against this disease via door-to-door campaigns (World Health Organization 2015). This international health intervention has faltered, however, with polio transmission persisting and US military actions contributing in part to this outcome.

On the surface, both polio eradication and drone strikes are simple interventions, aiming to eliminate a perceived threat (poliovirus or militant fighters) with surgical precision. But in both cases, planners' dreams of a simple solution, represented in medical operations or medical metaphors, have been stymied by the complexities of context. And in both cases, these ostensibly narrow programs have had broad impacts. The US military's strategy of relying on drone strikes, particularly on the Pakistan side of the border, has not just led to civilian casualties, but has dragged the program aiming to end polio into the current conflict.

War with Drones

Few things have changed how wars are being fought over the past decade more than the rise of drone warfare. From a handful of drone attacks under the Bush administration, the US military under President Obama, taking advantage of improved surveillance technology, greatly increased the use of these weapons from an estimated fewer than five strikes a year in the mid-2000s to more than one hundred in Pakistan alone in 2010 (New America 2018). These attacks are representative of the US approach to the war on terror, one that attempts to target and eliminate individuals and small groups of fighters without adequately protecting civilians or understanding the wider implications for the surviving local population.

Drone strikes have great political appeal in the United States because they both limit US casualties in comparison with ground warfare and aid in covert military operations, often being used in support of small units instead of demanding large numbers of ground troops. The number of drone strikes has actually been lower in Afghanistan, where the United States has troops on the ground and a bilateral security arrangement in place, leading to more consultation between the US and Afghan militaries.[1] In Pakistan, where there are technically no US soldiers operating, but large amounts of US military aid and tacit agreement on the indirect use of force, drone strikes have become the US tool of choice.

These strikes are part of a long history of Western military intervention in the area. Three wars were fought between the British Empire and Afghanistan in the nineteenth and early twentieth centuries. The British Empire and, later, the Pakistani government militarized tribes in the area by arming select groups to defend the border and later supporting militants from the area in the war in Kashmir. The border between Afghanistan and what is now Pakistan, never demarcated and still disputed, has communities along both sides who maintain social and political ties and cross regularly.

The porous nature of the border, and the militarization of tribes in the area, were accentuated further when millions of refugees fled Soviet-occupied Afghanistan in the 1980s (Rubin 2002). Later, the failure of the initial US intervention to achieve what were often contradictory goals of state-building, counterinsurgency, and counterterrorism, allowed the conflict to grow and spread (Coburn 2016). Many Afghan fighters still take refuge in Pakistan, contributing to a growing insurgency on the Pakistani side of the border. This insurgency is further fueled by a combination of economic marginalization, religious rhetoric, often imported by transnational militant groups, and the long-term disenfranchisement by the Pakistani state, which has long neglected the area.

The Pakistani military has responded to the rise of a Taliban movement in Pakistan by ordering a series of military incursions into both FATA (the Federally Administered Tribal Areas) and KPK (Khyber Pakhtunkhwa), provinces on the Afghan border, over the past several years.[2] The United States has assisted the Pakistani military in these efforts, as well as dramatically increasing its use of drone strikes.[3]

The US government generally refuses to comment on drone strikes in Pakistan, but the attitudes that drove the significant increase in drone strikes in 2009 and 2010 are evident in a RAND report (Jones and Fair 2010). Among other things, the administration argued that the Pakistani military intervention had largely been unsuccessful at targeting insurgent leaders and had displaced millions, while US drone attacks, in contrast, had succeeded in taking out what the report calls several "high-value" targets (ibid., 125). The authors downplayed the number of civilian casualties in these strikes, concluding with the suggestion that: "The United States should continue to deepen cooperation with Pakistan on the use of unmanned aerial vehicles, including MQ-1 Predators,

MQ-9 Reapers, and future models. They are extremely useful for intelligence; surveillance; reconnaissance; and, occasionally, targeting militants" (127).

There are several problems with US military claims that drones actually reduce civilian casualties in comparison with more conventional military tactics. The first is the lack of complete or clear data on drone casualties, as journalists are often kept from reporting in the area of the attacks. US government officials also frequently count civilian bodies as those of militants. During one fifteen-month period, the CIA claimed there had been no civilian casualties in the area of drone strikes in Pakistan, while the Bureau of Investigative Journalism identified eighty-nine, including sixteen children (Ross 2015, 100).

Two of the more complete databases are organized by the Bureau of Investigative Journalism and the New America Foundation, both of which report much higher civilian casualty rates than the US government. As of July 4, 2018, the BIJ reported a total of between 2,515 and 4,026 killed, between 424 and 969 of whom were civilians, and between 171 and 209 of whom were children, in 430 strikes (Bureau of Investigative Journalism 2015). The New America Foundation reported 414 strikes with between 2,366 and 3,700 casualties (New America 2018). Others who have assessed the impact of drone strikes argue that even these numbers are underestimates. Daniel Byman of the Brookings Institution, for example, suggested that there may be closer to ten times as many civilian as militant deaths due to drone strikes (Byman 2009).

One of the issues is the use of what the US government has called signature strikes, or drone attacks that do not target specific identified individuals, but individuals who have patterns of activity thought to be correlated with militant activity (Williams 2013). Groups engaged in certain actions, like "driving toward a certain house or gathering under a certain tree in a particular village," may be killed (Bennis 2015, 52). This further distorts casualty numbers since the Obama administration considered all military-age men killed in strikes to be military targets and not civilians (Cohn 2015, 13). Other strategies, such as "double taps," when a follow-up strike comes shortly after the initial strike, target those attempting to assist the wounded, a group that may well include emergency responders (Ross 2015, 15). These various approaches have helped produce the high numbers of civilian casualties.

All of these practices, in addition to the regular presence of drones along the border area, promote the militarization of daily life for civilians there. Simple choices, such as whether to gather as a group for a funeral or whether to use a government hospital when ill, may suddenly have deadly consequences. The consequences of living under such tense and unstable conditions are poorly understood. Almost no research has been done on the psychological harm that these attacks cause, for local residents and scholars have only just begun to put these attacks into historical context (Reifer 2015; Tahir 2015).

Afghans who live in the border area described to the authors how this uncertainty has affected their everyday life and choices. One young man described hiding behind one of his family's cows that had just been killed by a rocket, unsure where the next one might come from. In some cases, attacks targeted individuals who had ties with the insurgency, but while visiting the Afghan side of the border, local leaders complained that other attacks seemed to have no logic to them and had not been made on known combatants.

During visits close to the border, it was clear that clinics in the region, which had been some of the few places women could go without male escorts, were considered increasingly risky since the Taliban viewed them as affiliated with the international presence. As fighting between the Taliban and US troops increased, uncertainty about the ability to harvest crops or simply avoid attacks drove many Afghan civilians toward larger cities away from the border, such as Gardez, Kandahar, and beyond. They settled in makeshift housing, which further exacerbated the country's health crisis by taxing the resources of already limited hospitals where long waits and limited facilities were the norm.

Much is unknown about the public health repercussions of such a state of continual warfare. What are the long-term effects of years of attacks that have no warning? How do attacks reshape the worldviews and health of survivors?

Crumbling Health Systems Amidst War

Khyber Teaching Hospital, Peshawar, Pakistan, 2007. The hospital-green paint is peeling from the dirty walls of the pediatric ward, which smells of disinfectant and illness. There are no windows, and the weak fluorescent light is not enough to completely illuminate the dingy hallway. The ward is packed with very sick children and their mothers, most wearing burqas pushed back to show their faces. The ward is crowded, several children sharing each cracked vinyl bed. One tiny girl has an awful cough, and an infant is screaming. The lights go out entirely, leaving us in complete blackness, and then a moment later the lights flicker back on with the generator; nobody flinches. There are no doctors or nurses anywhere on the ward.

What we do know is that armed conflict has had a long-term, serious impact on health services in both Pakistan and Afghanistan. In Afghanistan, in the long war between the Soviets and the then US- and Pakistani-backed militants, health facilities were neglected or destroyed. While militant groups received ample international funds for warmaking, international aid to rebuild or staff health facilities in times of relative peace was woefully inadequate. Displacement and economic insecurity also took their toll on Afghans. The effects on health were severe and far-reaching. In Afghanistan in 2002, before drone warfare really began, adult life expectancy was just forty-six years, and infant and child mortality were among the highest in the world (Bhutta 2002).

Pakistan has a different history, but its health systems too have been neglected as a result of militarization. The government spends just 3.5 percent of its total government budget on health, among the lowest of any country in the world. (The global average is 15 percent.) This is in part a result of conflict, including particularly Pakistan's ongoing dispute with India over the Kashmir region. Pakistan has poured resources into national defense, at the expense of sectors like education and health (Suleri 2013). The result is that Pakistan's health indicators lag behind other South Asian countries. According to WHO estimates, eighty-six of one thousand children in Pakistan die before they reach five years of age—compared to forty-one in Bangladesh and fifty-six in India. Health indicators are even worse in the border areas, where people often live far from government services (Tahir 2015). Most of these deaths are preventable and treatable, from causes such as diarrhea, pneumonia, and relatively simple birth complications.

The current struggle to end polio is deeply affected by this history. If Pakistan and Afghanistan had strong health systems with good rates of routine immunization, polio would have long ago disappeared from those countries. But because their health systems often do not provide basic services like childhood vaccines, especially to the poor and marginalized, polio can gain a foothold.

In addition to these baseline problems, the current conflict provides further protection for the poliovirus.

The Campaigns to End Polio

Karachi, Pakistan, 2012. On this first day of the weeklong polio campaign, female workers, mostly in their teens and early twenties, arrive at the health post around 9 a.m. Most wear green polio eradication baseball caps on top of their black hijab. They sign forms and pick up their blue containers full of vaccine in a buzz of preparation. After a lot of waiting, they crowd into the back of a small Suzuki van that will deliver them to the areas where they will distribute vaccines.

Most of the teams of workers go door to door delivering polio vaccine. At each house, they'll record the number of children under five, giving vaccine to those children who are there and marking the house for follow-up if some are missing. Other teams of workers roam bus stations and markets, finding and vaccinating children in these public places.

Pakistan and Afghanistan, along with Nigeria, are the only countries in the world where the Global Polio Eradication Initiative has failed to ever eliminate polio. With the goal of stamping out the virus completely, eradicators have instituted an intense program of vaccination across both countries. In the border areas of Afghanistan and Pakistan, there has been a weeklong door-to-door polio campaign nearly every month for the past ten years. As many as ten times a year, houses in these areas are visited by vaccinators hired by the government who are attempting to find and vaccinate every child under five. Many children have been vaccinated against polio as many as thirty or forty times.[4] In part these repeated campaigns are necessary because the oral polio vaccine has low efficacy in places where many children have enteric infections. But polio transmission continues because there are some children who are still under-vaccinated, either because they are repeatedly missed by the campaign teams or because their parents refuse the vaccine for their children.

Unfortunately, the campaign may represent the only health services a family gets. Focused exclusively on eliminating polio, these campaigns usually do not provide other health services, frustrating families who might desperately need obstetric care for a high-risk pregnancy, or medicine for someone dying of tuberculosis. It is often impossible to get these services from neglected government health facilities, particularly along the border. But that same government health system brings polio vaccinators repeatedly to their doorstep.

This stark difference between polio services received and other health services received has two causes. One is the low levels of government funding for health, discussed above. The other is the heavy international focus on polio, which receives hundreds of millions of dollars a year in separate streams of international funding. An international official in Islamabad explained in 2012, "There is huge involvement of the donor community [in polio].... Bill Gates himself is calling the president... Truly speaking the government doesn't spend anything for polio.... WHO, the World Bank, UNICEF and JICA are funding it" (Closser et al. 2014).

International actors are committed to polio eradication for several reasons. First, and most significantly, the prospect of being part of a historic initiative ending a disease forever is a motivator for donors like the Gates Foundation and Rotary International, who lobby governments to give as well. In addition, eradicating polio would mean that governments could eventually stop vaccinating their own populations against the disease, resulting in long-term financial benefits (Taylor, Cutts, and Taylor 1997), one reason that the US government finances polio eradication both through USAID and the CDC.

The Campaign against the Campaign

Rawalpindi, Pakistan, 2007. In a dusty vacant lot between crowded apartment buildings, a henna-bearded grandfather had pulled a *charpoy* [wood-and-rope cot] into the sunshine. He sat there playing with his granddaughter, who was about a year old. When I [SC] approached, he immediately and correctly assumed that I was affiliated with polio eradication. As I walked toward him, he said in Urdu, "We don't give polio drops to our children. It's my right to bring them up in the way I think is best."

I agreed that this was indeed his right, and he added that he didn't want to give his children anything "unIslamic." I started to ask why he felt polio drops were unIslamic, but was interrupted by a government health supervisor who had seen us talking and come to see what was going on. He told the grandfather sternly, "This memsahib[5] was so worried about your granddaughter that she came all the way from America to immunize her. And you don't care enough about your grandchildren to let her do it?"

This, predictably, set the grandfather off. "America drops bombs on us Muslims but then says they are sending vaccines to *help* us?"

This man was critiquing international actors' claims of beneficence in the overall context of war. It is not surprising that people with reason to be suspicious of their governments—given ongoing military operations in their area—would begin to worry that a vaccination campaign is not what it seems (Closser et al. 2016). For many parents, these fears were exacerbated when the CIA used a fake hepatitis B vaccination campaign to confirm the identities of Osama bin Laden's family members (Aikins 2013; Saeed 2011). Widely publicized accounts of this operation made fears that vaccination campaigns were actually in service to US military surveillance seem more plausible.

The GPEI's polio public relations campaigns have historically downplayed the political dimensions of suspicions about vaccination campaigns. Insurgent leaders, meanwhile, have used uncertainties around polio campaigns to their advantage. In 2012, the Pakistani Taliban banned polio campaigns in North Waziristan, an area of Pakistan near the border with Afghanistan (Ahmad, Bux, and Yousuf 2015). A fatwa (religious decree) banning campaigns, written by cleric Hafiz Gul Bahadur, stated that polio campaigns would not be allowed in the area until drone strikes were stopped.

The fatwa cited several reasons for this position. First, it criticized international priorities, arguing that the negative health impacts of drone strikes far outweighed the health impacts of polio: "Polio infects one child in a million, but hundreds of Waziri women, children and elders have been killed in these strikes," the fatwa said, adding, "Each day the list of psychological patients increases in Waziristan, which is worse than polio" (Nasruminallah 2012). The fatwa further notes that polio campaigns might be a way for the United States to spy on locals.

In short, the fatwa both legitimated and reinforced local fears about and resentments of polio campaigns. The ban on vaccination remained in place until June 2014, when a Pakistan military intervention brought these areas more securely back into government hands, with the side effect of allowing polio vaccination to resume.

Bahadur's fatwa was followed by declarations by other scholars and leaders on both sides of the border in opposition to polio campaigns (Gul 2012). Bahadur is not simply, as is sometimes stated, part of the Pakistani Taliban. Rather, Bahadur is very much a product of the past decades of military conflict in the frontier region, which have led to the decline of tribal leaders and figures who could simultaneously maintain connections with the militant groups, tribal elders, and the government. These hybrid leaders draw on a variety of sources for their legitimacy, from their tribal backgrounds to their ability to attract international funds. As a result, these figures look at issues like polio campaigns pragmatically, using them as a part of wider political projects and bargaining.

Bahadur is not alone in attempting to refuse polio campaigns in order to gain concessions from the Pakistani state or international actors. His fatwa emerges from a longer history of so-called demand refusals—when communities refuse polio vaccine wholesale, not because they are opposed to vaccination per se, but because they are protesting what they see as the misplaced priorities of governments and international organizations. Communities refuse polio vaccines in protest over lack of electricity, sanitation, and other health services such as medication for common illnesses. They attempt to use the obvious importance of polio eradication to international and national officials as a route to services that they more urgently need. Communities in Pakistan in general, and in the border areas in particular, have tried this tactic sporadically, and usually on a small scale, since at least 2005.

Negotiating using such refusals has not usually worked, however, both because polio eradication officials resist the pressure, and because they usually do not have control over the other services that citizens so desperately need. As far as drones specifically are concerned, the head of polio eradication at WHO claimed that locals "know we don't have any control over drone strikes" (McNeil 2012).

But while nearly all polio eradication officials, in Pakistan and internationally, are opposed to drone strikes, for many locals they are linked:

Both are interventions by the government, in collaboration with foreign agencies and governments, which are disconnected from or antithetical to quite urgent local needs. Local leaders have been able to use polio activities as a symbol of the government's disconnection from its citizens' desires, sowing fears about a disease control project in the process.

The Health Worker Murders

Because polio eradication is an obvious priority of international actors and the Pakistani government, and because health workers are so visible in local communities, they have become an attractive target for insurgents. Starting in December 2012, militants began murdering the local health staff going door-to-door delivering polio vaccine. Over the next three years, they murdered at least thirty and perhaps as many as eighty polio workers in Pakistan (World Health Organization 2015).

The campaign workers—mostly women—are not highly paid aid workers. They do not have ties to international interests. They are people who take very low-paid work for polio campaigns, often earning just a few dollars a day, in an attempt to support their families and help their neighbors. Insurgent leaders know this. So why are they targeting the workers?

It is likely that insurgents have several aims in these coordinated attacks against health workers. Because polio eradication is such a high-profile project, and because ground-level workers are relatively vulnerable, it is an easy way to attract international attention (Abimbola, Malik, and Mansoor 2013). The fact that international agencies and the government have loudly announced their commitment to the eradication of polio probably contributed to the symbolic value of the project— and its workers—as representative of both Pakistani government and foreign, including US, interests (Closser and Jooma 2013).

In Afghanistan, the Taliban has sometimes supported polio campaigns, and sometimes opposed them, depending on where their political interests lie. The various branches of the Taliban in Afghanistan have shifted their approach toward polio vaccination programs, first allowing these projects to operate in Taliban-controlled areas, later attacking health workers, then calling these attacks off again (Abimbola et al. 2013; Stancati 2014). Notably, one of the main reasons they gave for attacking healthcare workers was the fact that they were accused of spying for international actors. Whether or not Taliban leaders actually thought that local health workers were spying for foreign governments, the high visibility of polio eradication made it an attractive symbolic target.

Insurgent groups' competition with one another also influences these attacks. The rise of Daesh, the Afghan branch of the Islamic State, in part stemmed from widespread sentiments among local commanders and their troops that the Taliban had failed to expel international troops from the country. During 2015, there were initial negotiations between Taliban leaders and Afghan officials despite the Taliban having long suggested that they would not engage in such dialogues until all American troops had left the country. This suggested to some that the Taliban was perhaps not as committed in their opposition to the Afghan government as they claimed to be. Unsurprisingly, then, in 2015, Daesh prevented polio campaigns in several districts in Nangarhar, a clear attempt to enhance their credentials as opponents of drone strikes and the international presence more generally (Sahil 2015).

Polio on the Rise

Currently, Afghanistan and Pakistan are the last countries in the world that have not been able to stop polio transmission. In 2014, Pakistan had 328 cases of polio, the highest in years; Afghanistan had 28 cases. The majority of the cases in Pakistan were in the border areas with Afghanistan. Many of the cases in Afghanistan were from poliovirus that came from Pakistan, perhaps carried by migrants fleeing the ongoing conflict there. Since 2012, the vast majority of polio cases have been in areas where militants are attacking health workers and some parents are refusing vaccines for reasons related to drone warfare.

Areas where children are inaccessible to vaccinators because of conflict or bans on polio vaccine are a particular challenge for polio eradicators. In 2013, more than 500,000 children were inaccessible in Pakistan, and another half million were sporadically inaccessible in Afghanistan. Polio eradication's leadership reports a "very close correlation between areas of inaccessibility, location of cases, and areas of low population immunity" (Global Polio Eradication Initiative 2015).

A recent study (SteelFisher et al. 2015) provides some insight into the specific effects that conflict has on polio vaccination. In higher-conflict areas of Pakistan, only 70 percent of parents surveyed said that their children had received polio vaccine in the last campaign (a percentage likely too low to eliminate the virus); in lower-conflict areas, in contrast, 93 percent of parents surveyed said that their child had gotten vaccinated. At least a third of parents in higher-conflict areas believed at least one negative rumor about polio vaccine (for example, that the vaccine caused sterility in children) compared to only 12 percent of parents in lower-conflict areas. And parents in higher-conflict areas trusted polio vaccination workers less.

While drone strikes have made the project of ending polio more difficult, they are not the sole cause of polio cases. They exacerbate preexisting problems, such as people's dissatisfaction with the government health system for its failure to deliver many essential services. The central reason for that distrust is the government's long neglect of health provision, a problem tied to decades of conflict. And some children are under-vaccinated simply because teams do not visit their homes as planned. A lack of good pay and support to the lowest-level workers is a factor as well.

But the ongoing armed conflict makes the effort to end polio that much more complex and means that simply running more and more campaigns might actually undermine attempts at eradication. In the context of international interventions like drone strikes, polio eradication's repeated door-to-door campaigns focusing on just one relatively rare disease are more likely to seem suspicious and offensive to parents. For those living on the border, it is difficult to simply separate military and health aspects of the ongoing conflict.

A War with and without Borders

The US argument for using drone warfare includes the claim that it produces fewer casualties, both military and civilian. This calculus, however, ignores the wider impacts of such targeted attacks. The example of polio shows that drone attacks have politicized health interventions, eroding confidence in health programming and ultimately contributing to the deaths of more civilians. Polio transmission is evidence of the broad and diffuse health effects of war: It is an indirect result of war's impacts on both health systems and political rights in Afghanistan's and Pakistan's conflict zones (Mazzarino, Inhorn, and Lutz, this volume).

On the surface, both polio eradication campaigns and drone strikes are surgically narrow programs that planners can imagine have few effects beyond their targeted activities. But no military or health intervention exists in a vacuum. These two programs, planned and implemented by very different groups of international actors and Pakistani government officials, have become entangled on the ground. The resulting civilian deaths are in addition to the contested counts of those people killed directly in drone strikes. They include, among many others, a young female Pakistani health worker, murdered as she vaccinated children in an Afghani refugee camp on March 16, 2015, and a seven-month-old boy in North Waziristan, paralyzed by polio on May 6, 2015. The legacy of distrust and the imbalance in healthcare efforts that contributed to these civilian casualties is likely to remain long after drone strikes end.

Acknowledgments

This chapter includes interview and fieldnote data collected by Sarwat Jehan, Patricia Omidian, and Emma Varley.

NOTES

1. See the reports cited for more precise numbers (Bureau of Investigative Journalism 2015; New America 2015).
2. The Pakistani Taliban is independent of, but deeply linked to, the Afghan Taliban.
3. The Pakistani Taliban, the Afghan Taliban, the Haqqani Network, and numerous other smaller groups along the border all have slightly different goals and ties with international jihadi groups like al Qaeda. For the most part, however, ties to these international groups tend to be overstated and most concerns are deeply local, which is part of what gives these groups their symbiosis (see Bergen and Tiedemann 2012).
4. While this is a lot of vaccination, there are no significant known risks or side effects from receiving a large number of doses of oral polio vaccine (OPV). OPV is generally very safe; the major risk to the vaccinated child is getting polio from the vaccine itself (called "vaccine associated polio paralysis" or VAPP). There is not strong evidence that a large number of doses of OPV increases the risk of VAPP to a given child (Platt, Estívariz, and Sutter 2014). In general, ensuring population immunity through mass vaccination prevents around 1,000 cases of wild polio for

every case of VAPP it causes, making vaccination well worth the small risk. There is a current shift toward using fewer campaigns, not because of concerns about VAPP but because, as described in this chapter, repeatedly vaccinating the same children so many times can lead to community opposition.

5   A female honorific used primarily for white women, with strong colonial overtones.

REFERENCES

Abimbola, S., A. U. Malik, and G. F. Mansoor. 2013. "The Final Push for Polio Eradication: Addressing the Challenge of Violence in Afghanistan, Pakistan, and Nigeria." *PLoS Med* 10(10): e1001529. doi.org/10.1371/journal.pmed.1001529.

Ahmad, S. O., A. S. Bux, and F. Yousuf. 2015. "Polio in Pakistan's North Waziristan." *The Lancet Global Health* 3(1): e15. doi.org/10.1016/S2214-109X(14)70353-5.

Aikins, M. 2013. "The Doctor, the CIA, and the Blood of Bin Laden." *GQ* (January). Retrieved from www.gq.com.

Bennis, P. 2015. "Drones and Assassination in the US's Permanent War." In *Drones and Targeted Killings: Legal, Moral and Geopolitical Issues*, edited by M. Cohn, 51–62. Northampton: Olive Branch Press.

Bergen, P., and K. Tiedemann. 2012. *Talibanistan: Negotiating the Borders Between Terror, Politics, and Religion*. Oxford: Oxford University Press.

Bhutta, Z. A. 2002. "Children of War: The Real Casualties of the Afghan Conflict." *BMJ* 324(7333): 349–52. doi.org/10.1136/bmj.324.7333.349.

Bureau of Investigative Journalism. 2018. "Drone Strikes in Pakistan." Retrieved from www.thebureauinvestigates.com.

Byman, D. 2009. "Do Targeted Killings Work?" Brookings Institution, July 14. Retrieved from www.brookings.edu.

Closser, S., K. Cox, T. M. Parris, R. M. Landis, J. Justice, R. Gopinath, . . . E. Nuttall. 2014. "The Impact of Polio Eradication on Routine Immunization and Primary Health Care: A Mixed-Methods Study." *Journal of Infectious Diseases* 210(suppl 1): S504–S513. doi.org/10.1093/infdis/jit232.

Closser, S., and R. Jooma. 2013. "Why We Must Provide Better Support for Pakistan's Female Frontline Health Workers." *PLoS Med* 10(10): e1001528. doi.org/10.1371/journal.pmed.1001528.

Closser, S., R. Jooma, E. Varley, N. Qayyum, S. Rodrigues, A. Sarwar, and P. A. Omidian. 2016. "Polio Eradication and Health Systems in Karachi: Vaccine Refusals in Context." *Global Health Communication* 1(1): 1–9. doi.org/10.1080/23762004.2016.1178563.

Coburn, N. 2016. *Losing Afghanistan: An Obituary for the Intervention*. Stanford, CA: Stanford University Press.

Cohn, M. 2015. "Introduction: A Frightening New Way of War." In *Drones and Targeted Killings: Legal, Moral and Geopolitical Issues*, edited by M. Cohn. Northampton: Olive Branch Press.

Crawford, Neta. 2018. "Human Cost of the Post-9/11 Wars: Lethality and the Need for Transparency." Costs of War Project. Retrieved from http://watson.brown.edu/costsofwar/.

Global Polio Eradication Initiative. 2015. *Global Polio Eradication Initiative (GPEI) Status Report*. London: GPEI. Retrieved from www.polioeradication.org.

Gul, P. 2012. "North Waziristan Tribes Lose Perks for Not Supporting Anti-Polio Drive." *Dawn*, December 17.

Jones, S. G., and C. C. Fair. 2010. *Counterinsurgency in Pakistan*. Santa Monica, CA: RAND Corporation. Retrieved from www.rand.org.

McNeil, D. 2012. C.I.A. "Vaccine Ruse in Pakistan May Have Harmed Polio Fight." *New York Times*, July 9. Retrieved from www.nytimes.com.

Nasruminallah. 2012. "No Polio Drives in N Waziristan unless Drone Strikes Stop: Hafiz Gul Bahadur." *Express Tribune*, June 16.

New America. 2018. "Drone Strikes: Pakistan." Retrieved from www.newamerica.org.

Platt, L. R., C. F. Estívariz, and R. W. Sutter. 2014. "Vaccine-Associated Paralytic Poliomyelitis: A Review of the Epidemiology and Estimation of the Global Burden." *Journal of Infectious Diseases* 210(suppl 1): S380–S389. doi.org/10.1093/infdis/jiu184.

Reifer, T. 2015. "A Global Assassination Program." In *Drones and Targeted Killings: Legal, Moral and Geopolitical Issues*, edited by M. Cohn, 79–90. Northampton: Olive Branch Press.

Ross, A. 2015. "Documenting Civilian Casualties." In *Drones and Targeted Killings: Legal, Moral and Geopolitical Issues*, edited by M. Cohn, 99–131. Northampton: Olive Branch Press.

Rubin, B. R. 2002. *The Fragmentation of Afghanistan: State Formation and Collapse in the International System*. New Haven, CT: Yale University Press.

Saeed, S. 2011. "CIA Organized Fake Vaccination Drive to Get Osama bin Laden's Family DNA." *Guardian*, July 11.

Sahil, M. 2015. "Daesh Prevents Polio Campaign in Three Nangarhar Districts." *Tolo News*, October 10.

Stancati, M. 2014. "Afghan Taliban Bans Polio Vaccination in Southern Province." *Wall Street Journal*, July 7.

SteelFisher, G. K., R. J. Blendon, S. Guirguis, A. Brulé, N. Lasala-Blanco, M. Coleman, . . . C. Sahm. 2015. "Threats to Polio Eradication in High-Conflict Areas in Pakistan and Nigeria: A Polling Study of Caregivers of Children Younger than 5 Years." *Lancet Infectious Diseases* 15(10): 1183–92. doi.org/10.1016/S1473-3099(15)00178-4.

Suleri, A. Q. 2013. "Insecurity Breeds Insecurity." In *Development Challenges Confronting Pakistan*, edited by A. M. Weiss and S. G. Khattak, 57–69. Sterling, VA: Kumarian Press.

Tahir, Madiha. 2015. "Bombing Pakistan: How Colonial Legacy Sustains American Drones." Retrieved from http://watson.brown.edu/costsofwar.

Taylor, C. E., F. Cutts, and M. E. Taylor. 1997. "Ethical Dilemmas in Current Planning for Polio Eradication." *American Journal of Public Health* 87(6): 922–25.

Williams, B. G. 2013. "Inside the Murky World of 'Signature Strikes' and the Killing of Americans with Drones." *Huffington Post*, March 31.

World Health Organization. 2015. *Summary Report on the Technical Consultation on Polio Eradication in Pakistan* (No. WHO-EM/POL/414/E). Cairo: WHO Regional Office for the Eastern Mediterranean.

3

Remaining Undone

Heroin in the Time of Serial War

ANILA DAULATZAI

It was June 2011. I was in the last months of more than four years of anthropological research with widows and their families in Kabul, Afghanistan, when I was introduced to Aisha by Marium, a widow in her fifties whom I had come to know quite well. Marium and I had just traversed the congested city center, and she began giving more specific directions to the driver as we approached an informal settlement of houses in the southwest of the city. Leaving the car, Marium knocked on a metal door and asked if Aisha was home. We were directed to a large one-room structure on the left side of an open courtyard, where Aisha greeted us. She had been living there for four years, sharing the space with her son and two other widows, as well as their three children. We small-talked as Aisha's son served us green tea and biscuits. Marium recalled how they had met almost eight years earlier while they were both standing in line to receive their monthly rations in an aid distribution program that supported vulnerable widows. Since then, Aisha and she had become good friends.

Aisha was in her mid-thirties when we met. She had been widowed five years earlier, but she had been receiving rations from an aid program for widows for three years prior to actually losing her husband. The aid program nonetheless had classified Aisha as a widow because her husband was listed as *mayub* (disabled) in documents testified by their neighborhood *wakil* (legal representative) and certified by the Afghan Ministry of Martyrs and Social Welfare. Disabilities have become commonplace in Afghanistan as a result of decades of serial war, and Afghans distinguish between people born with disabilities and others who become disabled as a consequence of some sort of misfortune in the course of their lives. *Mahlul* is a term usually used to refer to a person born without disability, but who became disabled—usually a result of missing limbs, etc. *Mayub* is usually used to refer to someone born with a disability, or with a disability of unknown origin and/or where the person's body appears intact but does not function as expected. There is some flexibility, overlap, and contestation, however, between the colloquial uses of *mayub* and *mahlul*. As *mayub* is also used for disabilities of unknown origin or reason, some consider drug users *mayub*, and not *mahlul*. Such contestations are an example of the ways Afghans have had to respond to the range of conditions that serial war produces on their bodies, and how institutions and individuals respond to this range of disabilities. Aisha's husband was considered disabled because he had been an active drug user until his death. Aisha had thus been able to obtain rations as a widow due to *mayubiat*, her husband's condition of dependency on heroin. Aisha was thus de jure a widow because she was a woman whose husband was incapacitated and unable to economically provide for her.[1]

After her husband's passing, Aisha continued to receive rations from the aid program. However, within a year after her husband's death from a heroin overdose, and about five years before our first meeting, Aisha began using heroin herself and stopped going to the monthly distributions to get rations.

In our conversations, Aisha repeatedly stated that while her husband was still alive, she had never been interested in using heroin together with him.

> I only started using after he left this world. I could not take care of our son, who was seven years old at the time of his father's death. I just wanted to sleep all the time. After my husband had died, his friends and others would visit and bring me prepared food to help me and my son. I started using heroin after a friend of my husband's came to bring us some food and firewood for winter. I asked him if heroin would help my condition. Since then, I am using heroin every day.

Aisha had two sons. One of them died in a bomb blast on his way to school when he was eight years old. Her husband had been walking with her son, and even though the husband was injured in the blast, he survived.

After the *jinazah* (Islamic burial) of our son, my husband stopped talking for a few days. A few more days later, he started using heroin and said it allowed him not to feel pain anymore. He used heroin every day until he died, five years ago. So you tell me Anila, what killed my husband? Heroin? The death of our son? This *haalat* (condition, situation) that is Afghanistan, all of this, all of this killed both of them, and it will probably kill me, too.

Much important research on Afghanistan focuses on the drug trade or, specifically, the heroin economy as part of the networks that operate alongside and within the war economy. Much crucial public health work on heroin users in Afghanistan focuses on HIV, risk behaviors, harm-reduction strategies, and clinical classifications for mental illness (Todd et al. 2005; Kuo et al. 2006; Todd, Abed., et al. 2009; Todd, Stibich, et al. 2009; MacDonald 2008; Maguet and Majeed 2010; Saif ur-Rehman et al. 2007; Starkey 2009; Tschakarjan and Vogel 2009; UNODC 2003, 2005, 2009; Sherman et al. 2005; Ahmed et al. 2003; Haque et al. 2004; Strathdee et al. 2003; Zafar et al. 2003; Hankins et al. 2002; Vogel et al. 2012; Zafar and ul Hassan 2002). While risks posed by the spread of HIV and the links of heroin use with mental illness are certainly critical issues that need to be addressed in concrete ways in Afghanistan, no ethnographic studies exist that contextualize the predicaments of individual heroin users in Afghanistan and help to understand how such users are embedded in local worlds.

In the following, I will try to offer such an ethnographic reflection by focusing on the role of heroin in Aisha's life. There are two important points about Aisha to note at the outset. First, as already mentioned, she could not say what caused her husband's death. Was it heroin? Or was it the bomb blast that killed her son, and in so doing, created the conditions of possibility for her husband to turn toward heroin? Rather than answering any of these questions, Aisha refers to the *haalat*—the general conditions or situation—of her country as the reason for the deaths of her son and her husband. And second, this *haalat*, or condition, that constitutes contemporary Afghanistan includes roadside bombs and a military occupation, but also includes what I refer to as serial war, i.e., the current wars that are fought in the country (the so-called War on Terror, including the Taliban and more recently IS, but also the War on Drugs, and a War on Polio²) and those that came before and alongside it: the Soviet Occupation (1978–1989); the years of violence and upheaval following the Soviet Occupation, which I term the Kabul Wars (1989–1995); the Taliban rule (1995–2001); and the ongoing NATO-led invasion and occupation beginning in 2001 (as part of a "Global War on Terror"), all of which intersect in the lives and life trajectories of Afghans I have met in Kabul.

An important claim my research, in general, makes is that although these wars (the War on Drugs, the War on Terror, and the War on Polio) have distinct names, and have seemingly distinct temporalities, they should not be perceived as unrelated. Of course, certain connections are easily acknowledged, for example, how the Soviet Occupation created the conditions of possibility for the Kabul Wars that followed. Similarly, the CIA's funding and arming of specific groups in Afghanistan and Pakistan during the Soviet Occupation created the Taliban, which then created the conditions of possibility for the NATO-led invasion of 2001, the inaugural act of the ongoing Global War on Terror. However, while the genealogies and connections between the Soviet Occupation, the Kabul Wars, and the War on Terror are widely accepted, linkages between the distinctly named contemporary wars in Afghanistan and Pakistan (the wars on terror, on drugs, and on polio) are not commonly acknowledged. But what would it mean, analytically, to remove the distinct names assigned to these wars and to think of them as instantiations of the differing ways that serial war has marked the region since the late 1970s? If we consider that polio remains endemic in Afghanistan and Pakistan because of serial war, then we no longer see the war on polio simply as a public health campaign to eradicate a single disease. Instead, we recognize the presence of polio as a result of the seriality of war in the region, and thus, the militarization of a disease.³ Thinking in terms of serial war is precisely Aisha's point—to consider the *haalat* of Afghanistan, rather than isolated causal relations. When we are made to see things as discrete, separate, and unconnected (her husband's struggle with heroin and/or a polio-stricken child elsewhere in Afghanistan), it becomes too easy not only to render them as individual pathologies with established etiologies ("addiction," "polio," "roadside bombing"), but more importantly, to remove any necessity to interrogate the seriality of war and the ways these wars are connected, causally related, and dependent on one another, and entangled in the lives of Afghans.

Furthermore, reflecting on the bomb blast itself, Aisha makes no clear distinction between the physical pain her husband faced from the injuries he sustained in the blast that killed her son, and the psychic pain of a father having to see his son killed in front of him. In our conversations, I tried to distinguish the psychic pain from the injuries, but Aisha was clear on not wanting to privilege one pain over the other, or to attribute his turn to heroin to physical pain. He was in pain, and he used heroin to treat that pain. As I will show, the story of how heroin entered Aisha's family life and stayed there allows us to see how serial war resides in the lives and life-making potentials of Afghans.

In a 2013 volume with the same name, Eugene Raikhel and William Garriott introduced the concept of *addiction trajectories*: "In highlighting the notion of trajectories, we aim to emphasize the directed (yet contingent) movement of people, substances, ideas, techniques, and institutions along spatial, temporal, social, and epistemic dimensions" (2013). Garriott and Raikhel continue by articulating three specific addiction trajectories: the epistemic, the therapeutic, and the experiential. I would like to borrow from Garriot and Raikhel in thinking about *heroin trajectories* and focus on experiential trajectories of lives and subjectivities in relation to serial war and heroin in Kabul, and beyond. What role does heroin play in recuperating or enabling alternate forms of life, or modes of living that are not life-affirming, in contrast to modes of life imagined and articulated (if not exclusively) by liberal forms of thought and modes of intervention? How does the *haalat* (condition, situation) of serial war in Afghanistan build up to form intimacies with heroin such that the substance is enfolded into lives as forms of kinship and world belonging?[4] In saying this, I do not mean that people only form such intimacies with substances in contexts of serial war. I am instead asking what it would mean to take serial war analytically seriously along with the question of how these wars reside in the heroin trajectories of people like Aisha. In contrast to populations of drug users that have been studied elsewhere (Agar and Reisinger 2002; Bourgois 2003; Bourgois and Schonberg 2009; Garcia 2010; Garriot 2011; Goodfellow 2008; Reinarman and Levine 2004), it is not landscapes of poverty and/or racism that dominate the biographies of Afghan heroin users, but primarily the context of serial war (which, however, also entails poverty and racism).⁵ In both the logics and practices of state and non-state actors, serial war has, in the course of the past four decades, serially rendered Afghans killable. How may these logics and practices thus forge modes of living that may not necessarily tend toward vitality? How might they constitute a quest for a particular form of life and living that is not a non-attachment to life, but is an attachment to something somehow otherwise, yet nevertheless, resilient? Aisha's heroin use should not make us assume that she does not have an attachment to living or being alive, but that the modes of living life that she is expected to comply with simply do not align with her experience of being in the world. Elizabeth Povinelli, writing about aboriginal populations in Australia in the face of what she terms "late liberalism," asks: "Which forms of endurance will they find themselves inhabiting, the kind that makes them hardened, calloused, and indifferent to life or strengthens their attachment to life?" (Povinelli 2011, 116). In making parallel inquiries to Povinelli's, one may want to ask what makes Aisha—who lost a son, and then a husband to the *haalat* that is Afghanistan—turn to heroin while others in Afghanistan do not? I will deliberately not address this question because I learned from Aisha that it might be imbued with the imperative to assess which forms of resilience and endurance are to be valued and reified as the good life, the empowered life, and which ones are not. Rather, I will ask how we may understand Aisha's use of heroin not merely as a form of exhaustion, but as a mode of endurance and resilience in the face of truly exhausting conditions or circumstances.

Initially, Marium had been hesitant to introduce me to Aisha. As Marium explained, "She will perhaps give you a bad picture of widows in Afghanistan. Even after you have been here so long, Anila, I find it special that you still think you need to learn more about widows, you still want to understand more about their lives, and possibilities. This is why I want you to meet Aisha, but please understand, Anila, I also worry that she will give a bad image to you of widows." I mention Marium's hesitancy as it signaled to me an invitation to encounter a different way of being a widow, a different mode of life, perhaps, from what I had become accustomed to seeing thus far in Kabul. Marium mentioned the word "bad" at least four or five times during that particular conversation, and I was intrigued by what she might mean. I realized only after I came to know Aisha and to understand Marium's modes of care and her relationship to Aisha, that Marium did not mean "bad" in a judgmental or moralizing way. Rather, Marium used "bad" to index a mode of life that she thought I may be uncomfortable with, a mode of life that did not fit neatly into the imagination of the normative subject of liberal wars and humanitarianism, to which Afghans, especially those in Kabul, have become accustomed since the US-led occupation began in 2001. While Aisha's was thus not a mode of life Marium herself was uncomfortable with, she recognized it as one that would certainly be judged as "bad" from the perspective of liberal humanitarianism, and which would be a target for aid programs. Aisha's heroin use would certainly be a behavior that would be the target of reform in harm reduction programs, as heroin use is harmful. Furthermore, heroin use is certainly not a mode of life that is empowering to women—according not only to the logics of harm reduction, but to liberal feminist humanitarian logics in Afghanistan. What is often left out or completely unattended to in such programmatic logics of empowerment and self-improvement are the larger risks and harms posed by war. There are very few harm reduction programs that would target or even name war as a harm to be reduced, particularly in the context of drug use, as the narrative of addiction enables an exclusive focus on an individual pathology.

The aid distribution program run by CARE International (where Marium and Aisha had met and where I had also first met Marium) was the longest standing aid program for the most vulnerable widows of Kabul city. I came to know the project, the workers, and the beneficiaries quite well over the four years of my fieldwork. In 2008, after years of expanding their program for widows across districts in Kabul, CARE began to gradually reduce the number of widows who were receiving rations, and then later, began to aggressively implement programs to get widows to work as unskilled laborers. This was the NGO's way of thwarting what in aid programs and development parlance is referred to as "dependency." Marium eventually started working as a cleaner at Kabul University, as that was the only way she could continue to receive rations and a small salary. Aisha, however, decided she no longer wanted to receive rations from CARE after she began using heroin.

The ration distributions were a lively space of gossip and rumor. Monthly, widows were being dropped from the aid program for the slightest change in their circumstances. Often, the news that they were dropped was announced openly by the aid workers, which often was a rather messy and demeaning thing to witness for everyone involved, especially the widows. Elsewhere I have detailed the accusations of corruption and suspicion that were present between staff, widows, and others (Daulatzai 2013). The space of the ration distribution was then also often a place where people felt betrayed. While I point to the general anxieties around dependency that permeate aid and development discourse and practice, and to how the ration program for widows aimed to wean women off their dependency on handouts by making them work, as in Marium's case, there is a different axis around which dependency figures in relation to widows in these programs: Women need to be recognized as sufficiently vulnerable and dependent in the first place in order to qualify as a beneficiary in the program. CARE program staff used rigid institutional criteria to determine whom to include and exclude from future rations. Widows strategically deployed these criteria to assess one another as deserving or not, as they waited in line to receive their allotments. They gossiped over who really was deserving, often referring to the most vulnerable as *masakeen* (rightful recipients of care, according to the Quran). Thus, the ration distribution was a remarkably competitive and often unforgiving space.

When Aisha's husband was alive and he was declared *mayub* (disabled due to his dependency on heroin), Aisha felt that she would be judged for not being an actual widow, and that others might think she was taking away the right from a *masakeen*. Marium continually reassured Aisha that she never heard anyone speak of her in that way and added that she would have never allowed that in any case. A heroin user for the past five years, yet a widow who was deemed vulnerable enough to receive rations from CARE, Aisha felt she might be judged for her heroin use by other widows who were vying for a ration card. However, CARE would not necessarily know she was using heroin, and Marium reiterated that other widows at CARE certainly did not judge her for her heroin use. She was, thus, largely not judged for her heroin use outside of this particular context.

Aisha explained that she simply stopped going to get the rations. She was being cared for by friends and family, who brought enough food for her and her child-like Marium, who every month, without fail, shared her rations with Aisha. I witnessed such non-judgmental responses by Afghans to heroin users throughout my time in Afghanistan.

Instead, people described the woes the heroin user had faced in life that would cause them to succumb to the drug. When they were not speaking with the voice of the aid institutions some of them worked for, Afghans seemed to understand the proximity of heroin in their lives, largely as a consequence of the *haalat* that is Afghanistan. To cite one other example of this non-judgmental response, I was at a vegetable stall later that week, buying some fruits and vegetables to take to Aisha. A man who was clearly a heroin user passed the stall, with his head hung low. The vegetable seller hastily filled a plastic bag with assorted fruits, ran, and handed them to the stranger. He came back and under his breath said: "Sister, aren't we all only half a step away from being *tariyaki* (someone who uses heroin or opium)." Ordinary Afghans understand the vulnerabilities that result from serial war, and moreover, the contemporary contingencies that make us all vulnerable, albeit differently, at any point to a turn to heroin. The compassion, or *shafaqat*, that Afghans enact for fellow Afghans is a far more relevant obligation in Kabul nowadays with regard to heroin than Islam's prohibition of intoxicants. The unconditional and non-judgmental compassion that Aisha receives is indicative of one of the ways ordinary Afghans respond to the turns that a life can take, living amidst the *haalat* that is Afghanistan. Aisha has a steady flow of friends, like Marium, who consistently bring her food, medicines, and other necessities.

Aisha's clarity in stating that she does not know how to name what killed her husband—heroin, or the violence that killed her son (and that made her husband turn to heroin)—should make us want to know what may be at stake for others who exclusively say that it was heroin that killed her husband. Since her husband's death, friends, heroin rehabilitation case workers, and countless others put pressure on Aisha to enroll in one of Kabul City's heroin rehabilitation clinics. Aisha told me that when heroin rehabilitation case workers refer to her husband's death, they attribute it to heroin. Similarly, while political analysts, security analysts, drug policy researchers, and others have done important work on Afghanistan's contribution to the global heroin epidemic (as opposed to heroin that remains in Afghanistan), they also have a singular focus on heroin. Yet in choosing not to attend to the *haalat*, as

Aisha instructs us to do, at least two problems ensue. First, when the focus is on an individual pathology or on what is commonly referred to as "addiction" in biomedical approaches to heroin use, we risk fetishizing the substance while simultaneously allowing for moral anxieties created during the War on Drugs to eclipse modes of relationality between substance and user that fall outside typical addiction paradigms.[6] Second, when we identify heroin as that which killed Aisha's husband, we simply fail to take serial war analytically seriously. I do not only refer to the ways that histories of drugs converge with histories of wars in very critical and revelatory ways in Afghanistan. Taking account of war necessitates a shift in attention away from substance use and toward the experiential aspect of living amidst serial war, and to what Afghans are subjected to as well as responsive to. Critically engaging with Aisha would mean taking seriously the subjective trajectories of heroin users in Afghanistan and their particular relation to serial war. It means considering how wars and occupations allow for intimacies with heroin while steadfastly resisting any temptation to abstract heroin and the Drug War in Afghanistan from the greater *haalat*.

Aisha accepted care daily from friends and neighbors who, like Marium, visited her frequently and unconditionally to check on her and her son, and to bring food or other necessities. However, Aisha was quite confident in her decision to discontinue receiving rations from CARE, even though she was entitled to them, and even though she still had a current ration card, a highly sought-after asset among widows in Kabul. It is important to consider what might be at stake in Aisha's refusal. She knew that Marium and other widows now had to participate in job trainings or work programs in order to receive their monthly rations. Yet Aisha was not refusing because of the prospect of having to work, although her heroin use might have posed a challenge in performing certain work duties. Instead, Aisha refused to comply with the specific range of expectations the training and work programs implied: that she should become empowered (as a widow) or rehabilitated (as a heroin addict). She simply refused to perform the role of the good widow or the good ex-heroin user.

Much emphasis of the international intervention in Afghanistan, particularly the humanitarian and development discourses of the past fifteen years, has centered on liberal imaginations of empowered women (particularly, but not exclusively, widows). In such a framework, there is a very explicit need to demonstrate that women are self-sufficient and independent. Such programs credit themselves and the international community who enacts them, together with the resilience of the women themselves, for their proclaimed success. Elsewhere I have written on neoliberalism, not only as a form of economic restructuring, but as a social form or a form of governmentality that cultivates neoliberal subjects in Kabul (Daulatzai 2015). I explored the ways neoliberalism has become embedded in everyday life in Kabul such that social relationships and obligations to widows have been reconfigured. I looked specifically at the mandate to get widows to work in Kabul as a way to thwart aid world anxieties around "dependence" and to simultaneously cultivate a form of agency (or sovereignty over the self) that cannot materialize under conditions of occupation, as is the case in Afghanistan.

CARE and similar international and national organizations have focused on the economic development of individual widows, thus constructing imaginaries of what a successfully empowered Afghan widow should look like. While opportunities offered to widows by CARE (and others) have certainly altered their lives for the better, it is critical to reflect on who may be excluded from these possibilities on offer, such as women like Aisha. Aisha refuses rations from the organization not only because she fears they may be conditional on her not using heroin, but relatedly, because she also does not want to submit to liberal humanitarianism's image of what an Afghan widow should or must be doing, in her case, as related to heroin. She does not feel it appropriate that widows, and others, who choose to use heroin to endure their days should only be encouraged to work or enroll in heroin rehabilitation programs. In returning to the quote offered by Povinelli, articulating a form of life being "otherwise": "Which forms of endurance will they find themselves inhabiting, the kind that makes them hardened, calloused, and indifferent to life or strengthens their attachment to life?" (Povinelli 2011, 116). Aisha does not inhabit a form of endurance that is hardened or calloused, nor one that is strengthening an attachment to life, yet neither is she particularly attached to death. Rather, she shows an attachment to a life differently articulated.

Thinking alongside Aisha and her heroin use trajectory has allowed for an exploration of a less comfortable mode of living life in a war zone. There is sufficient writing that explores the resilience of women in spaces of war and violence, demonstrating the ways that women make do in the most violent and exhausting of circumstances (Liebling-Kalifani 2010; Radan 2007; Ryan 2015; Wanga-Odhiambo 2014). These are accounts of women who persevere in ways we now have come to expect them to persevere in, always. Such a focus on resilience demonstrates the "agency" that women have, the ways they creatively craft their lives and the lives of others amidst very difficult circumstances. Women labeled as resilient are to perform productivity, and to recover from prior harm. While such a focus on resilience is important in countering representations of women as passive victims who are being acted upon, it is ultimately unaccepting of a subject infinitely marked by violence, of a body that does not recover, or of a self that refuses to recover. Sarah Bracke explores the cultivation of resilience as a neoliberal value, as what she refers to as a "regime of resilience" (Bracke 2016, 14). While neoliberal modes of governance are certainly relevant in the case of Afghanistan, I am here raising the problem posed by the cultivation of particular normative modes of resilience in the face of serial war. Resilience regimes, thus understood, allow simultaneously for a de-politicizing of the forces that necessitate resilience—in the case of Aisha, the *haalat* of Afghanistan. Furthermore, regimes of resilience sanitize and exclude more unsettling and distressing modes of resilience. Aisha and her family compel us to take account of a less comfortable mode of life, an account that destabilizes normative imaginations of what Afghans—as widows, or heroin users, or as heroin-using widows—need or should be doing as resilient subjects of violence and serial war. Thus, this chapter should be read as not only about the current phase of war in Afghanistan, but about serial war, attending to the durational aspects of what war does and the general *haalat* created by serial war for individuals, families, and communities. Marium, who was widowed in another era of serial war than Aisha was widowed, cares for Aisha and Aisha's son alongside the obligations Marium has to her own family. New forms of kinship and relationality are forged in war. I am acknowledging only two here (while many more can and must be explored): kinship formed between two widows, Marium and Aisha, and between Aisha and the substance heroin.

One afternoon, Marium and I visited Aisha. It had been a tough week for Marium as she was being trained in a new livelihood program. She wanted to spend the afternoon with Aisha and make sure Aisha was okay. Marium worried when she was unable to check in with Aisha twice a week, in person or by mobile phone, and this week had been far too hectic for her. When we sat together at Aisha's, Marium began telling us how the NGOs running the economic development trainings she was undergoing often resort to treating widows like idiots who would be unable to manage their lives without the ingenuity of such programs and the care of the international community. Aisha turned to me and said, "This is why Marium and I are such good friends, she does not judge me when I use heroin, and I do not judge her when she does whatever the organizations want her to do to be a good widow." Marium nodded in agreement: "They do work hard to make sure we know how important it is that we do not become dependent and that we get jobs. I am not sure how it happened, but I find myself continuing to do what they want us to do as now I am dependent in a different way than I was before—dependent on the salary, and because I depend on the rations to be able to share them with Aisha." Not only is Aisha refusing to submit to the logics and practices of the aid regimes of care, but Aisha is asking us to consider ways of being resilient that do not fit within the regimes of resilience manufactured by institutionalized imaginations of care present in contemporary Kabul.

Bracke articulates what she refers to as a "hegemonic ethos of resilience": "Don't mourn too hard, too long, too loud; or too dangerously. Don't be undone, and don't undo. Bounce back. Take the impact—the fire, the heat, the suffocation—and bounce back. To your original shape, if you can" (Bracke 2016, 11). In deliberately remaining undone, Aisha is articulating another way of being resilient. Despite the normative expectations of resilience permeating the regimes of care of the international intervention in Afghanistan, Aisha encourages us to make room in our analyses for modes of life that do not fit the images of an empowered Afghan widow, or a rehabilitating heroin user, or an empowered, rehabilitating Afghan widow heroin user. Aisha does all this, and more, as she also refuses to let us crudely understand heroin as that which killed her husband, asking us instead to consider the *haalat* of Afghanistan—serial war that created the conditions of possibility for her husband, and now her, to be resilient yet otherwise resilient.

NOTES

1 Elsewhere I have written on the ways Afghan women creatively work with aid program classifications to allow those falling outside of criteria to become classificatorily widowed in order to receive access to much needed material assistance (Daulatzai 2006).
2 In contrast to the "War on Drugs" and the "Global War on Terror," which are phrases officially deployed by US governments, the expression "War on Polio" emerges from the discursive spaces of journalism and global health, which embrace the same language of securitization and militarization while referring to public health campaigns aimed at eradicating the disease (Bhutta 2013; Bill and Melinda Gates Foundation 2011; International Crisis Group 2015; Kennedy, McKee, and King 2015; Rogers 2014; Saifee 2016; Sherazee and Ebrahim 2015).
3 How polio eradication campaigns are related to serial war in the region is the focus of my ongoing research in Pakistan.
4 I take up the relationship between heroin as a form of kinship elsewhere "Substance and Kinship in Kabul: Heroin in the time of Serial War" (Daulatzai 2017).
5 This is not to say that landscapes of poverty and racism in the United States, for example, are not also constituted by structures of violence of a serial nature.
6 Writing about alcohol and indigeneity in India, Roger Begrich shows that the relation a user may have to a substance (such as alcohol in the case he describes, or heroin in the case discussed here) may only be one particular relationship among a wide range of relationships that matter in that person's life. If that relationship between substance and user is diagnosed as *addiction*, other relationships become eclipsed. Begrich thus offers a critique of the addiction paradigm by thinking about such relations between substances and humans in terms of obligations (2013, 2017).

REFERENCES

Agar, Michael, and Heather Schacht Reisinger. 2002. "A Heroin Epidemic at the Intersection of Histories: The 1960s Epidemic among African Americans in Baltimore." *Medical Anthropology* 21 (2): 115–56.

Ahmed, Mohammad Abrar, Tariq Zafar, Heena Brahmbhatt, Ghazanfar Imam, Salman ul Hassan, Joseph C. Bareta, and Steffanie A. Strathdee. 2003. "HIV/AIDS Risk Behaviors and Correlates of Injection Drug Use among Drug Users in Pakistan." *Journal of Urban Health* 80 (2): 321–29.

Begrich, Roger. 2013. "Inebriety and Indigeneity: The Moral Governance of Adivasis and Alcohol in Jharkhand, India." PhD diss., Department of Anthropology, Johns Hopkins University.

———. 2017. "Drinking as Obligation. An Anthropological Critique of Addiction." Unpublished manuscript.

Bhutta, Zulfiqar A. 2013. "Conflict and Polio: Winning the Polio Wars." *JAMA* 310 (9): 905–06.

Bill and Melinda Gates Foundation. 2011. Polio Eradication: A Must-Win Battle in the Global War on Disease. Bill and Melinda Gates Foundation, Global Health Program. Retrieved from docs.gatesfoundation.org.

Bourgois, Philippe. 2003. *In Search of Respect: Selling Crack in El Barrio*. Cambridge: Cambridge University Press.

Bourgois, Philippe I., and Jeffrey Schonberg. 2009. *Righteous Dopefiend*. Berkeley: University of California Press.

Bracke, Sarah. 2016. "Is the Subaltern Resilient? Notes on Agency and Neoliberal Subjects." *Cultural Studies* 30 (5): 1–17.

Daulatzai, Anila. 2006. "Acknowledging Afghanistan: Notes and Queries on an Occupation." *Cultural Dynamics* 18 (3): 293–311.

———. 2013. "Flows of Suspicion: Corruption and Kinship in Kabul, Afghanistan." In *Local Politics in Afghanistan: A Century of Intervention in Social Order*, edited by Conrad J. Schetter. New York: Columbia University Press.

———. 2015. "What Does Work Mean to Widows in Afghanistan?" *Harvard Divinity Bulletin*, 43 (1 and 2).

———. 2017. "Substance and Kinship in Kabul: Heroin in the Time of Serial War." Unpublished manuscript.

Garcia, Angela. 2010. *The Pastoral Clinic: Addiction and Dispossession along the Rio Grande*. Berkeley: University of California Press.

Garriott, William. 2011. *Policing Methamphetamine: Narcopolitics in Rural America*. New York: NYU Press.

Goodfellow, Aaron. 2008. "Pharmaceutical Intimacy: Sex, Death, and Methamphetamine." *Home Cultures* 5 (3): 271–300.

Hankins, Catherine A., Samuel R. Friedman, Tariq Zafar, and Steffanie A. Strathdee. 2002. "Transmission and Prevention of HIV and Sexually Transmitted Infections in War Settings: Implications for Current and Future Armed Conflicts." *Journal of the International AIDS Society* 16 (17): 2245–52.

Haque, N., T. Zafar, H. Brahmbhatt, G. Imam, S. ul Hassan, and S. A. Strathdee. 2004. "High-Risk Sexual Behaviours among Drug Users in Pakistan: Implications for Prevention of STDs and HIV/AIDS." *International Journal of STD and AIDS* 15 (9): 601–07.

International Crisis Group. 2015. *Winning the War on Polio in Pakistan*. Asia Report No. 273. Retrieved from www.crisisgroup.org.

Kennedy, Jonathan, Martin McKee, and Lawrence King. 2015. "Islamist Insurgency and the War against Polio: A Cross-National Analysis of the Political Determinants of Polio." *Globalization and Health* 11 (40). doi: 10.1186/s12992-015-0123-y.

Kuo, I., S. ul-Hasan, N. Galai, D. Thomas, T. Zafar, M. Ahmed, and S. Strathdee. 2006. "High HCV Seroprevalence and HIV Drug Use Risk Behaviors among Injection Drug Users in Pakistan." *Harm Reduction Journal* 3 (26).

Liebling-Kalifani, Helen. 2010. "Research and Intervention with Women War Survivors in Uganda: Resilience and Suffering as the Consequences of War." In *War, Medicine and Gender: The Sociology and Anthropology of Structural Suffering*, edited by H. Bradby and G. Lewando-Hundt. Farnham Surrey: Ashgate Books.

Macdonald, David. 2008. *Afghanistan's Hidden Drug Problem: The Misuse of Psychotropics*. Afghanistan Research and Evaluation Unit (AREU).

Maguet, O., and M. Majeed. 2010. "Implementing Harm Reduction for Heroin Users in Afghanistan." *International Journal of Drug Policy* 21: 119–21.

Povinelli, Elizabeth A. 2011. *Economies of Abandonment: Social Belonging and Endurance in Late Liberalism*. Durham, NC: Duke University Press.

Radan, A. 2007. "Exposure to Violence and Expressions of Resilience in Central American Women Survivors of War." *Journal of Aggression, Maltreatment and Trauma* 14 (1–2): 147–64.

Raikhel, Eugene, and William Garriott. 2013. "Addiction Trajectories: Tracing New Paths in the Anthropology of Addiction." In *Addiction Trajectories*, edited by Eugene Raikhel and William Garriott. Durham, NC: Duke University Press.

Reinarman, Craig, and Harry G. Levine. 2004. "Crack in the Rearview Mirror: Deconstructing Drug War Mythology." *Social Justice* 31 (1–2): 182–99.

Rogers, Naomi. 2014. *Polio Wars: Sister Elizabeth Kenny and the Golden Age of American Medicine*. Oxford: Oxford University Press.

Ryan, Caitlin. 2015. "Everyday Resilience as Resistance: Palestinian Women Practicing *Sumud*." *International Political Sociology* 9 (4): 299–315.

Saifee, Jessica. 2016. "The War on Polio." *Huffington Post*, April 8. Retrieved from www.huffingtonpost.com.

Saif-ur-Rehman, Mohammad Zafar Rasoul, Alex Wodak, Mariam Claeson, Jed Friedman, and Ghulam Dastagir Sayed. 2007. "Responding to HIV in Afghanistan." *The Lancet* 370 (9605): 2167–69.

Sherazee, Mahnoor, and Zofeen Ebrahim. 2015. "War on Polio: Is It All Spiraling Out of Control for Pakistan?" *Dawn*, June 6. Retrieved from www.dawn.com.

Sherman, S., S. Plitt, S. ul Hassan, Y. Cheng, and T. Zafar. 2005. "Drug Use, Street Survival, and Risk Behaviors among Street Children in Lahore, Pakistan." *Journal of Urban Health* 82 (3 Suppl. 4): iv113–24.

Starkey, J. 2009. "Afghanistan's Forgotten Heroin Addicts." *Asian Development Bank Publication* 5.

Strathdee, Steffanie A., Tariq Zafar, Heena Brahmbhatt, Ahmed Baksh, and Salman ul Hassan. 2003. "Rise in Needle Sharing among Injection Drug Users in Pakistan During the Afghanistan War." *Drug and Alcohol Dependence* 71 (1): 17–24.

Todd, Catherine S., Abdullah M. S. Abed, Paul T. Scott, Naqibullah Safi, Kenneth C. Earhart, and Steffanie A. Strathdee. 2009. "A Cross-Sectional Assessment of Utilization of Addiction Treatment among Injection Drug Users in Kabul, Afghanistan." *Substance Use and Misuse* 44: 416–30.

Todd, Catherine S., Naqibullah Safi, and Steffanie A. Strathdee. 2005. "Drug Use and Harm Reduction in Afghanistan." *Harm Reduction Journal* 2: 13.

Todd, Catherine S., Mark A. Stibich, M. Raza Stanekzai, M. Zafar Rasuli, Shairshah Bayan, Saifur Rehman Wardak, and Steffanie A. Strathdee. 2009. "A Qualitative Assessment of Injection Drug Use and Harm Reduction Programmes in Kabul, Afghanistan: 2007." *International Journal of Drug Policy* 20 (2): 111–20.

Tschakarjan, S., and M. Vogel. 2009. "Pilot Mental Health Assessment in Injecting and Non-Injecting Heroin Drug Users in Kabul, Afghanistan: A Semi-Structured Interview with 30 DU Visiting Regularly the MdM DIC in Kabul, Afghanistan." Unpublished manuscript.

United Nations Office on Drugs and Crime (UNODC). 2003. *An Assessment of Problem Drug Use in Kabul City*. Kabul: United Nations Office on Drugs and Crime.

———. 2005. *Afghanistan Drug Use Survey*. Vienna-Kabul: United Nations Office on Drugs and Crime.

———. 2009. *Afghanistan Opium Survey 2009*. Vienna-Kabul: United Nations Office on Drugs and Crime.

Vogel, Marc, Senop Tschakarjan, Olivier Maguet, Olivier Vandecasteele, Till Kinkel, and Kenneth Dürsteler-MacFarland. 2012. "Mental Health among Opiate Users in Kabul: A Pilot Study from the Medecins du Monde Harm Reduction Programme." *Intervention* 10 (2): 146–55.

Wanga-Odhiambo, Godriver. 2014. *Resilience in South Sudanese Women: Hope for Daughters of the Nile*. Plymouth, UK: Lexington Books.

Zafar, Tariq, Heena Brahmbhatt, Ghazanfar Imam, Salman ul Hassan, and Steffanie A. Strathdee. 2003. "HIV Knowledge and Risk Behaviors among Pakistani and Afghani Drug Users in Quetta, Pakistan." *Journal of Acquired Immune Deficiency Syndromes* 32(4): 394–98.

Zafar, Tariq, and Salman ul Hassan. 2002. "A Sociodemographic and Behavioral Profile of Heroin Users and the Risk Environment in Quetta, Pakistan." *International Journal of Drug Policy* 13 (2): 121–25.

4

Dignity under Extreme Duress

The Moral and Emotional Landscape of Local Humanitarian Workers in the Afghan-Pakistan Border Areas

PATRICIA OMIDIAN AND CATHERINE PANTER-BRICK

The threat of kidnapping, beheading, and bloodletting is now part of the landscape of humanitarian aid in the border areas of Afghanistan and Pakistan. Let us begin with one concrete example. In January 2013, one of the headlines of the Pakistan edition of the *International Tribune* read: "Swabi bloodletting: In grisly attack, gunmen kill seven aid workers" (Express Tribune, 2013). Two attackers, riding a motorcycle, intercepted the van transporting staff from a non-governmental organization (*Support With Working Solution*) working in Khyber Pakhtunkhwa province. They pulled a five-year-old child away from his mother before spraying the vehicle with bullets, killing one man and six women, all local Pakistani workers delivering health and education in the region. In speaking to the press, the NGO director described the crux of the tragedy, from a local perspective, in these terms: "The innocent girls worked to support their families." This example situates humanitarian practice in the context of militant violence and states of emergency, articulates the dangers and dire tension that *local* humanitarian aid workers confront because of their profession, and highlights their predicament in having assumed humanitarian work to guarantee their families' livelihood.

Targeted killings of local aid workers, such as the January 2013 attack, have profound consequences on both NGO and government employees who develop and manage the delivery of health and other services. For example, the killings of nine polio fieldworkers, shot dead in a string of attacks in Karachi and border towns in December 2012, prompted the government of Pakistan to suspend the polio eradication campaign in many areas of the country, and forced WHO and UNICEF to withdraw their technical and monitoring personnel; despite all political efforts and increased resources, the eradication campaign could not be implemented in areas where polio was most prevalent. Targeted killings also have critical health and social consequences for the local staff who work as technicians, health workers, teachers, translators, or drivers for government and humanitarian agencies. Until recently, we have known more about the front-line stories of expatriate aid workers (Bergman 2003; Orbinski 2008; Redfield 2012; Ager and Iacovou 2014), than the circumstances of local aid workers, in terms of the risks they undertake to provide for their families and the dilemmas they face with heightened insecurity. Unlike their expatriate counterparts, local aid workers, often employed by small NGOs, have few safety nets and travel with little or no protection (Omidian 2001, 2011). They are called upon to provide services within their own communities, often eliciting local jealousy and resentment. They may be internally displaced persons (IDPs) themselves. As we illustrate in this chapter, even those employed by government agencies are placed at risk; in the humanitarian business, no one is now exempt from death threats.

One recent appraisal of the systematic harassment of health workers described the situation in northern districts of Pakistan as follows: "The Taliban had launched a systematic campaign of abuse and harassment of the primary healthcare programme and its core workforce. . . . They used a combination of *fatwas* (religious decrees), threats, and physical assaults" (Ud Din, Mumtaz, and Ataullahjan 2012). These fatwas had serious implications for women community health workers, who "deliver services to the doorstep since societal norms restrict women's ability to attend healthcare facilities." Accordingly, one fatwa declared that the presence of women in public spaces was a form of public indecency, and that a Muslim man's duty was to kidnap female health workers when they paid home visits and marry them forcibly, even if they were already married; one Taliban chief stated it was acceptable to kill them. A second fatwa declared that it was morally illegal for Muslim women to work for wages. Daily radio programs were used to discredit female health workers, fueling encouragement to harass them (ibid.). It should be noted that many of the anti-government actors are often labeled as Taliban, even though they represent varied groups in the region, including the Taliban, Jihadists, and drug lords, regardless of their background or affiliation. Such militant groups target Pakistani government and military representatives in this region, and by extension, local health workers, given that in Pakistan, much of humanitarian aid is delivered through the operation of local government. Thus, community health and humanitarian aid workers have to operate within a context of systematic harassment and routine threats of violence, facing the same dangers as government employees such as police or security personnel.

A History of War and Insurgency

The area of Pakistan that borders on Afghanistan, inclusive of Khyber Pakhtunkhwa (KP, formerly called the Northwest Frontier Province of Pakistan), the Federally Administered Tribal Areas (FATA), and Baluchistan, is especially dangerous and violent. This region has been undergoing a rapid transformation, as border areas shudder under the weight of war and violence—drone attacks by the United States, fighting between the Pakistani army and the Pakistani faction of the Taliban, and killings by local war or drug lords. More than thirty local aid workers were killed or kidnapped in these areas in 2012 alone. These were men and women employed by agencies of the provincial government, delivering health and education services in the conflict zones or in the IDP camps established within FATA and KP.

The targeted killing of government employees involved in the delivery of humanitarian aid or reconstruction effort has roots in the recent history of Pakistan/Afghanistan relations. Pakistan had hosted one of the largest single refugee populations in the world: Afghans fled their country during the war against the Soviet-backed regime (1979–1989), with another surge of refugees during the period of civil war when the Taliban gained control of most of Afghanistan. At that time, Pakistan also supported the Taliban and other insurgent groups. With the attacks on the World Trade Center in 2001, the United States led a coalition of international forces to launch new military operations. The Taliban forces reverted to an insurgency campaign, now in its second decade. This war has brought into stark relief the weaknesses of Pakistani military support, given its tolerance for radical groups—often no more than drug or gun runners operating under a guise of Islamic rhetoric, connected to groups that Pakistan supported to fight against the Indian army along its joint border in Kashmir. Government and insurgent groups are engaged in a long, drawn-out battle over the strategic control of these regions.

Unfortunately for Pakistan, the support of militants along its two borders has brought about major instability in a country traditionally tolerant of diversity. Pakistan is now a deeply divided nation struggling to contain and curtail radical militants within its own borders, even as it tries to maintain pressure on Afghanistan. The methods used by the Taliban and other insurgents in Afghanistan, including selective assassination of government workers, military personnel, and civilians, are now common in Pakistan. Many of the insurgent groups take action against high-profile health campaigns to maintain pressure on the Pakistani government. In the midst of all this upheaval and complex politics, humanitarian work comes under duress, as targeted harm is inflicted to those who deliver healthcare and other forms of assistance.

Reflections on Humanitarianism in Action

In this chapter, we reflect upon the narratives of local humanitarian aid workers and the concerns of organizations delivering humanitarian aid locally. Our material is drawn primarily from group discussions and face-to-face interviews held during training workshops in Islamabad, funded by UN Women at the request of the Government of Pakistan's FATA Secretariat—specifically, its Women Empowerment Wing in the Social Sector, a department within the provincial government that administers social welfare, health, and humanitarian assistance in the tribal areas. We provide reflections on medical humanitarianism in action, at both personal and institutional levels, through the lens of the personal narratives of local humanitarians and through the lens of institutional training practices and policy concerns.

First, we highlight the dilemmas faced by local humanitarians, individuals who put themselves and/or their families at great personal risk because of their involvement with local and international humanitarian organizations. We provide ethnographic context to understand their situation, convey their psychological distress, and articulate the many different reasons for pursuing this type of work in the face of such grave danger. This gives voice to "what really matters" when living a moral life amidst uncertainty or danger (Kleinman 2006). It helps us reflect on what dimensions of emotional and social experience will make everyday life possible under the threat of targeted killings. We touch upon expressions of suffering, precariousness, and extreme duress, as well as the cultural straitjacket on public displays of emotion. We also reveal expressions of resilience and human dignity, articulated by the significance of a moral calling. As described in the narratives of ordinary men and women in neighboring Afghanistan, a strong sense of resilience to adversity is anchored in cultural values of faith, honor, moral code, service, perseverance, and family unity (Eggerman and Panter-Brick 2010). Such values promote a sense of coherence about life: namely, a sense that one's life is worth something, a sense of responsibility to one's family and community, and a sense of moral and social respectability. In this cultural context, resilience means more than an individual's ability to cope with adversity: It means holding onto a narrative of life that coalesces psychosocial well-being with collective notions of social justice, social worth, and social responsibility (Panter-Brick 2014).

Second, we reflect on the value of training workshops, capturing the complexities of life inside humanitarian spaces. Such a workshop, using a person-centered psychology approach known as *Focusing* (Gendlin 1982), served two institutional purposes. It provided psychosocial training to humanitarian staff working for local government or NGO agencies to alleviate distress, fear, and burnout. It also served to develop materials for humanitarian staff and beneficiaries, such as a training manual to be published in two local Pakhtu dialects for use during future workshops in IDP camps within FATA and KP areas. Our case study included twenty-two participants (twelve women, ten men), invited by the FATA Secretariat from a range of border areas (Malakand, Bajour, Mohmand, Khyber, Orakzai, and Waziristan), all of which experienced poor health services and very low literacy rates. They came to the workshop for a period of four weeks, both to cope with their work-related stress and to articulate what might be useful in the creation of a manual designed to assist the agencies' beneficiaries.

Living a Life under Extreme Duress

During the workshop, the extreme psychological distress participants experienced soon became evident. Each person had a tale of extreme danger to tell: direct threats received or instances where colleagues had been killed, kidnapped, or threatened. One young woman working in a social welfare capacity within FATA whispered that her brother-in-law had recently been kidnapped. Her whole family was waiting to hear from the kidnappers regarding the ransom demand, hoping that he had been kidnapped for money and not by the Taliban, who would more likely kill him because he worked for the Pakistani government. The family also worried about this woman's own safety, given the nature of her employment and her movements along roads within tribal areas. Another aid worker recounted that his cousin had been killed on his way home from his office in Peshawar. His killers were never identified; while the police in Peshawar blamed the victim, saying it must have been the result of an enmity between rival family members, no one in the family could believe this. A third government worker gave this account:

> I have been threatened several times by religious extremists and I regularly receive threatening calls from unknown numbers. Our project staff was attacked several times as they went about their work. In 2011, one of our colleagues was killed in the FATA area, and another was abducted—he is still in captivity, after two years.

Most participants stated they took some form of tranquilizers to help them sleep at night, to control their stress, and to help hide their fear; though they were only in their twenties and thirties, they experienced headaches, generalized body pain, sleep disturbances and nightmares, stomach problems, and high blood pressure. Most expressed their gratitude: Although they were under a great deal of stress, they had homes and families to return to at the end of each day. Many found their work to be not only dangerous but also frustrating and distressing. In IDP camps, for example, conditions were grim, in that tents did not suffice to protect people from scorching hot summers or freezing winters, and the humanitarian services provided were extremely limited.

Why did humanitarian aid workers continue to work in this field, facing serious threats of kidnapping or assassination? One woman, trained in public administration and public health in emergency settings, had taken up her position out of a desire to serve her community; she continued her work because to stop would mean abandoning people in dire need. She felt a personal responsibility to give "service" to her community and country, this being her duty as a citizen and as a Muslim. Another program officer, who "thought of quitting" in the wake of repeated threats, expressed both relative powerlessness given his "very limited choices" for livelihood in Peshawar and a dignified stance to fulfilling a moral duty: "I believe in what I am doing, so I think I will stick to what I am doing."

Three Personal Narratives

We focus on three narratives to give ethnographic substance to the concerns, fears, and motives of humanitarian workers and to the moral calling that permeates everyday life with necessary dignity. Our interlocutors gave verbal informed consent to reproduce their stories; we changed their names and omit mention of their employing agency to preserve anonymity.

Our first narrative exemplifies the concerns of humanitarian workers who delivered humanitarian aid to IDP camps catering to Pakistani communities in the wake of armed conflict. Barialai worked in Jalozai Camp, one of the largest IDP camps near Peshawar. This site had originally been designated for Afghan refugees; in the 1980s, it was a very large "village-like" settlement, with adobe brick homes, shops, and clinics. To hasten the repatriation of these refugees to Afghanistan, the settlement was dismantled by the Pakistani government—and bulldozed to the ground, just before war broke out in Swat/Malakand in 2007–2009. The site was newly designated to house IDPs from within Pakistan but strictly limited to tents rather than permanent dwellings. The camp now hosts approximately 12,500 families from FATA areas. As recounted by Barialai:

> A few years ago all the [Afghan] refugees were finally expelled from the camp. UNHCR [the UN High Commissioner for Refugees] and other UN agencies were told by the Pakistan government to make sure there was nothing left of the camps; so the Afghans took their roofing poles and some even took their building stones. Clinics were dismantled and all the equipment taken away. The tube wells were removed and the whole area was bulldozed. The government gave the land back to the villagers who

had originally owned it. But within six months after the final destruction of the last of the houses, the war in FATA and the north started and IDPs began to arrive in large numbers from Malakand. The [Pakistani] government had to scramble. They got the land back from the villages on a lease and allowed the IDPs to start settling on it. But there were new rules. No one was allowed to build a wall, enclosure or building. Only tents were allowed. The government wants to make sure there are no permanent structures. Where the Afghan refugees had been able to make their camps into villages and replace their tents with permanent and weatherproof structures, the Pakistani IDPs are forced to survive the extreme heat of summer and the freezing winter temperatures in tents.

Barialai noted that people are suspicious of him because he is from the area but works for an international organization. He is resentful of the fact that Afghan refugees, who used to live in this camp, had better standards of living compared to the conditions his own people are now forced to live in. He feels shame and frustration at the government's policies toward Pakistani IDPs, but at the same time thanks Allah that his own family does not have to struggle in that way. He has received threatening phone calls and has attended the funerals of friends (fellow humanitarian aid workers) who were murdered. Threats hang heavy over him, but this is the only job he knows that can provide for his family, allowing his children to attend private schools and have a comfortable life. He draws on a sense of moral capital, which gives meaning to his life and provides consolation: Working with people who are suffering helps to sustain him through pain and fear, and seeing the dire conditions that exist in the tribal areas and IDP camps makes him feel that he has no right to complain. Rather, he expresses gratitude for his situation.

The emotional downside comes with the cultural prohibition on expressing fear or even admitting to being afraid. Barialai can only privately share what he feels: In his words, he has a hard external shell that is the only thing the public can see. The day he witnessed a bomb blast in Peshawar, he acted strong and brave, telling people to have courage and focus on the upside (no one was killed or injured and only property was lost): "We, my colleagues and I, had to evacuate people from the area, in case there were other bombs that might go off. I had to pretend to be something I am not. All the while I was shaking inside, feeling fear that

I could never share. All I want is to go into a safe place where I can be what I am really like. I am a human being, not a Rambo. But if I show people my soft side, that is a worry."

Our second narrative highlights the fears and plight of local humanitarian workers during a kidnapping. Taimor was kidnapped and held prisoner for many months, until his family could buy his freedom with over a million Pakistani rupees. He and colleagues were taken hostage by a group claiming to be Taliban in an attack near his office; he works for a humanitarian aid organization on the outskirts of Peshawar. They were blindfolded and transported in the back of a truck for several hundred kilometers to the south, into FATA. Their captors often stopped for breaks; they bought the captives some juice to drink and asked if they wanted to eat but treated them roughly and pushed them around in such a way that the captives did not know if they would survive the ordeal. Once in FATA, the captors drove up to a house owned by a local thug, entered the building and killed the inhabitants, before transferring their hostages inside. Other captives joined the hostages over the course of their imprisonment. Taimor stated: "There were twenty-five personnel from law enforcement agencies with me while I was being detained by the Taliban. Two of them were severely wounded. I forgot my own suffering and gave them medical help by putting on bandages and when required changing them. . . . This boosted the morale for all of us."

Taimor believed he could be killed, either by Taliban militants or by US drones targeting the area. To this day, he shakes and breaks out in a sweat when he hears the sounds of jets or helicopters overhead.

Our third narrative illustrates the repercussions of such an ordeal on everyday family life. At the time of his kidnapping, Taimor was engaged to his cousin, Romeena, a university student. She called this period the most difficult time in her life; not only did she suffer, but it proved to be one more struggle to overcome in order to finally get married. She waited and waited for news—whether Taimor was still alive, where he might be, and how they might secure his release—and felt too weak to continue her studies. In her words: "It was a sudden shock for me and I spent those months in desperation, all the time praying, not going to classes at the university. And when Taimor was freed, I thanked Allah for His kindness. I feel I am honored with bravery and that I handled the situation with patience. Now I am happy to recover from that tragedy."

While Taimor was held captive, Romeena's family rallied around her: "My friends supported me and my neighbors visited to my house daily. They organized a *khatam* [reading of the Holy Quran] for me and they gave me strength and the power to stand. With the help of my community members I got such good support every day and they held me and helped me in my stress."

But this is not a "happily ever after" story. There are lingering consequences for Romeena and her family. She confided that Taimor has really changed since the kidnapping. These days, the family is terrified when he becomes violent and loses his temper. Romeena tries to have patience, but right now she has to deal with a violent husband. Within Pakhtun culture, she has few resources to help her cope with violence in the home. She searches for ways to help her husband curb his violent outbursts, which she says are the aftermath of trauma. Taimor himself does not feel right about his new level of violence.

Both Taimor and Romeena work for humanitarian organizations. When asked why, they say they want to succor others who so desperately need help. And when pressed, they admit that the pay is very good and they would not make as much money in other jobs. Taimor now has a different position in the provincial government, getting lower pay but better benefits, which include housing and a car. Because conflict between the government and local Taliban continues, he remains a potential target. Yet he sees himself as blessed: "After I got freed, I got back all that I had lost by the Grace of Allah, and now I am very happy. Our son and daughter go to good schools in Peshawar." The ability to choose the school their children can attend is one reason why the couple remains in the humanitarian arena. They gain decision-making power, as well as prestige, through "noble" work.

Humanitarian Training

We now turn to reflect on the training workshops—born of institutional concerns to address fear, restore well-being, and strengthen resilience in the face of mounting insecurity and danger. Our case exemplar was co-facilitated by Omidian, a US medical anthropologist resident in Afghanistan and Pakistan from 1997 to 2012, and a Pakistani humanitarian worker, who had attended training workshops following the

Kashmir earthquake of 2005 and had specifically requested that the FATA Secretariat sponsor similar initiatives in Khyber Pakhtunkhwa. The workshop was designed to provide an opportunity for a number of humanitarian workers to take a break, learn participatory training techniques, and work on personal issues.

The workshop built upon an ongoing program developed specifically for Afghans implemented in Kabul nine years earlier (Omidian and Papadopoulos 2003; Omidian and Lawrence 2007; Omidian 2012). It was evaluated in situ for its efficacy in emotional healing and cultural relevance (Frohböse 2010). Its modular and participative format allows participants to identify and develop culturally grounded and gender-sensitive approaches to address salient psychosocial issues, discuss resilience and the culture of emotions from local perspectives, and practice the mindfulness techniques of Focusing. The workshop provides opportunities for participants to identify positive exceptions to the norm of experiencing suffering and fear in everyday life through identifying people who manage to do well and adopt coping behaviors that are locally valued. This process of identifying "exception through exemplars" is akin to drawing power through the recognition of positive deviance (Pascale, Sternin, and Sternin 2010). The process of centering on the positive aspects of human experience connects well with cultural values, Islamic practices, and local Sufi traditions.

Focusing techniques have been developed over a decade of work in Afghanistan: More than 17,000 Afghans participated in school-based and community-based training programs in the decade between 2002 and 2011.

In its implementation with humanitarian staff, the adoption of participative techniques ran counter to the prevalent educational culture, a system that values social hierarchy and rote learning of absolute truth. Participants expected to be instructed on rights and wrongs. They were glad to actively engage in small group discussions and other endeavors, but would be silent during large group discussions, falling in line with a cultural tradition that emphasizes received answers rather than asking critical questions and practicing reflexive thinking. Participants had known they would draw concrete benefits from the workshop: Here was the time and place for a four-week respite from the dangers and fears encountered in the front lines of everyday humanitarian work. But little by little, they also found themselves engaged with its content: The program resonated with their own needs, and the emphasis on mindfulness was consonant with their traditions. As the following examples illustrate, the workshop provided a space for learning to negotiate troublesome emotions while articulating the significance of their moral calling.

Emotions and Resilience

In the workshop, participants discussed various ways of understanding emotions and resilience in the context of delivering humanitarian aid in the wake of armed conflict. In groups of four to six people, they discussed the range of emotions arising from this work. What became clear was that men were restricted with respect to emotional expression: They were not allowed to show fear, grief, love, or doubt, as this would bring shame on the man and his family. Only three emotions were available to men for public display: anger, jealousy, and hate. Furthermore, displaying anger was contingent on social status. When angry, a man cannot take action against someone of higher status but will use aggression against someone who has little power over him. And when afraid, a man is not able to admit fear and must instead react with anger or hate. One man categorically stated: "A man who is afraid would act violently, even shoot a gun at someone, then escape." Because many men experienced trouble sleeping at night, which often led to extreme tiredness, outbursts of anger and aggression were common outcomes. Relative to men, women were less constrained in public displays of emotion, especially love, fear, and sadness. Once married, however, they had to be very careful, as they lived with in-laws in extended family settings. After marriage, the straitjacket of emotional expression is captured by a local: "When a co-wife's son dies, a woman would weep on the outside, but laugh in her heart."

Humanitarian aid workers constantly negotiated a changing landscape of emotions for themselves, their clients, and their own family members. The burden of fear, in a culture that disdains the weakness of men, led men to internalize psychosocial stressors in ways that are toxic to well-being and that manifest explosive anger in unpredictable, violent outbursts. The burden of frustration and anger also weighed on women, who had few outlets to show such emotions.

As a counterpoint to this discourse on emotions, participants drew upon a discussion of resilience through the identification of specific exemplars in their locality. They identified types of resilience that encompassed personal, family, community, religious, and economic dimensions. Most participants felt that they could draw from a well of inner strength, which allowed them to continue to work. They stated that maintaining a firm belief in Allah and a sharp awareness of one's duties and responsibilities were some of the most important building blocks to nurture a capacity for resilience. In addition, remaining a loyal citizen of Pakistan and loyal to the government was articulated as an important notion of duty and service to the country, over and above duty and service to one's family.

Focusing through Culture, Islam, and Sufism

We detail two examples of Focusing practices implemented in this workshop to illustrate how they served to foster psychological strength and build social connections. The first practice is designed to help a person find a safe, quiet inner place in a visualization exercise that is meditative and healing. A facilitator proceeds to give quiet instructions to help participants relax and turn their awareness inward to "a safe place inside." This aligns with the Sufi notion that the inner world is greater than the outer world and that one comes close to Allah, the divine, when one turns inward. Participants are invited to think of a place that is calm and relaxing (a garden or a place in the mountains near a river) and imagine themselves sitting in that space as they breathe deeply. They are then asked to remember something in their lives for which they are grateful and to pay attention to how their body feels as they recall this.

This first step of Focusing thus aims to elicit feelings of calm and peace that can be anchored to a specific place, recalled with gratitude. The next step is designed to help people distance themselves emotionally from specific problems and envisage their resolution, through the analogy of handling each troubling issue as if it were "a guest in my life." For Pakhtuns, guests are highly valued: Welcome or unwanted, guests must be treated with respect, kindness, and courtesy. In Pakhtun society, most houses have a separate space (called a *hujra*) where guests (*meelma*) can be made comfortable without disturbing the inner sanctum and privacy of women in the home. The same imagery is used in the workshop: Emotional issues are likened to the "inner guests" of the mind and deliberately managed in a specific social space. Participants were asked to close their eyes and imagine themselves in their safe place—then move forward to a *hujra* where specific problems could be met in the same way that guests should be greeted, after which they would return to their sanctum for renewed peace and calm. One participant declared, "I have too many things that worry me and I cannot stay in the safe place," but found in the "guesthouse technique" a concrete way of making his worries less troublesome.

The second Focusing exercise involved a weighing scale and a handful of dried beans. One participant would enumerate all the problems he or she could think of, placing a bean for each problem on one side of the scale, then think of all the good things he or she could be thankful for, placing a bean for each one of those onto the other side of the scale. Other participants in the group would prompt the person with ideas of blessings for which one might be thankful. One woman could not find anything to be thankful for: She struggled with harassment at work and a mother afflicted by mental illness at home. In her case, the Focusing activity simply gave her the opportunity to safely express her emotions and frustrations within the group—prompting her to say that she now felt some "ease," in contrast to what she had been feeling during the previous months. Other participants reached the conclusion that the "good" in their lives far outweighed the "bad." Against all odds, the balance sheet of life tended to the positive. One man was delighted by this realization: "We spend so much time complaining about what we don't have and forget to thank Allah for everything he has given us. It is always more." Many participants felt inspired to write local sayings, poetry, and Quranic verses on sheets of paper and then pin them to the walls. One handwritten *hadith* (a saying of the Prophet) thus hung on the wall: "Indeed amazing are the affairs of a believer! They are all for his benefit. If he is granted ease of living he is thankful; and this is best for him. And if he is afflicted with a hardship, he perseveres; and this is best for him."

Conclusion

Humanitarian aid work in this region is very difficult, even in quieter times, because of the remoteness of this area and the conservative social norms of its population. With increasing threats to both local and international aid workers, and the deaths of so many in the Afghan-Pakistan border areas, it has become a profession of high stress and great danger. Workers, who are often seen as colluding with the Pakistani government and US policy in the region, face targeted attacks and the uncertainty of being at the wrong place at the wrong time; they are also vulnerable to bombings by insurgents/military forces, and drone attacks. In spite of such dangers, local people continue to work for agencies that channel humanitarian aid: They cite a moral calling, a religious duty, a family responsibility, and a social obligation of service to one's community or country as primary reasons to extend help to fellow countrymen and women. For some, this type of work is the only option available to support their families economically; even so, their profession is described as a calling that carries a high moral capital.

Human dignity is the key to resilience, previous ethnographic work in this region has shown: Specifically, the six cultural values of faith, perseverance, service, family unity, moral code, and honor constitute the bedrock of resilience in the face of extreme duress, misery, and violence (Eggerman and Panter-Brick 2010). Put simply, human dignity is manifested by perseverance and a notion of honorable service to one's family and community; it is both a sense of self-worth and social respectability. In Pakistan, as in Afghanistan, we encounter specific forms of cultural and economic entrapments: People are squeezed tightly between the cultural dictates that govern their behavior in public spaces and the economic dictates that compel them to provide for their family. Ordinary people hold onto their faith, work to secure a livelihood, and express gratitude for their situation, in order to retain personal and social dignity amidst a landscape of competing cultural and economic obligations. There is, nonetheless, a shrinking configuration of opportunities for the expression of human dignity, given persistent violent conflict, chaotic governance, economic instability, and widening social inequalities (Panter-Brick and Eggerman 2012). While "dignity" and "service" provide meaning and coherence to life, this does not mean that ordinary people doing extraordinary work do not experience fear, despair, or resignation. And while resilience is key to weathering the stresses inherent in humanitarian work, and the expression of human dignity is key to why local humanitarians feel able to face danger, it does not mean that dignity is easy to come by.

Extreme duress, long-standing suffering, and dignified resilience are facts of life in these Afghan-Pakistan border areas marred by poverty and violence. There is no ethical or logistical quick fix to such a difficult situation. The officials responsible for local governance struggle with the huge challenge of delivering social welfare, humanitarian aid, and immunization campaigns in these conflict-ridden areas. The FATA Secretariat took steps to address the enormous toll exerted on the physical, social, and emotional well-being of its humanitarian staff, seeking to develop culturally meaningful training sessions for men and women in their employment. They were driven, in part, by the desire to emulate global humanitarian practice, namely, workshops held in the wake of disasters to address mental health and psychosocial well-being, and the development of manuals as concrete "deliverables" to help with humanitarian activity. This desire was, however, tempered with a tangible concern to steer away from Western-style psychotherapy in favor of culturally grounded techniques to strengthen well-being.

Focusing techniques—similar to mindfulness techniques—explicitly drew upon locally meaningful practices: turning inward rather than outward, expressing gratitude and fortitude to Allah, embedding resilience in family and community service, and addressing toxic issues as one might greet unwanted guests. These techniques worked well in the context of a training workshop, where emphasis on spiritual practices to counteract fear or despair could be carried over in everyday life or practiced with a support group. Indeed, upon their return from the workshop, three participants developed a plan to introduce Focusing training sessions for women in the Jalozai IDP camp. In Afghanistan, where the program was originally developed, similar programs continue to be organized in formal and semi-formal ways, being endorsed by at least two NGOs more than a decade after they were first locally developed. The *Focusing* workshops have undoubtedly helped many men and women cope with extreme adversity with a greater measure of social and emotional composure, but from an institutional rather than a personal standpoint, they constitute only small steps toward meeting the needs of humanitarian workers for tangible professional support.

Our ethnography highlights the importance of understanding in greater depth not only the fears and dangers of humanitarian work, but also the culture of emotions, the wells of resilience, the moral and socioeconomic dimensions of human dignity, and the opportunities for institutions to take small but important steps toward managing the burden of violence in humanitarian settings. We have focused attention on the extreme duress of everyday life: Danger and pain stem from prominent threats of abduction and targeted killings, but also from the concerted efforts to uphold Pakhtun dictates of honor and service to family and community while navigating the cultural straitjacket of emotional expression. Highlighting humanitarian work as a moral calling is a way for local humanitarians to ascribe moral value and meaning to their experiences of extreme uncertainty, stress, and danger. But to infuse life with human dignity is a constant struggle: Tragedy, misery, and relative powerlessness are part and parcel of the humanitarian encounter in refugee camps and conflict zones, and institutional responses are limited or sketchy. Holding onto a sense of dignity is, in essence, an exercise of mindfulness: it is an ongoing effort to create spaces for calm and composed social behavior and, in the midst of fear and pain, to valorize faith, hope, and gratitude.

REFERENCES

Ager, A., and M. Iacovou. 2014. "The Public Discourse of Medical Humanitarians: Scripted Narratives from Expatriate Website Postings." *Social Science & Medicine* 120: 430–438.

Bergman, C., ed. 2003. *Another Day in Paradise: Front Line Stories from International Aid Workers.* London: Earthscan Publications.

Eggerman, M., and C. Panter-Brick. 2010. "Suffering, Hope, and Entrapment: Resilience and Cultural Values in Afghanistan." *Social Science & Medicine* 71(1): 71–83.

Express Tribune. 2013. "Swabi Bloodletting: In Grisly Attack, Gunmen Kill Seven Aid Workers." *Express Tribune*, January 2. Retrieved from http://tribune.com.pk.

Frohböse, A. 2010. "*Focusing* in Afghanistan. An Exploratory Study of a Coping-Strategy for Traumatized Communities." Master's thesis, submitted at the Carl von Ossietzky University of Oldenburg.

Gendlin, E. 1982. *Focusing*, 2nd ed. New York: Bantam Books.

Kleinman, A. 2006. *What Really Matters: Living a Moral Life Amisdst Uncertainty and Danger.* Oxford: Oxford University Press.

Omidian, P. A. 2001. "Afghan Aid Workers and Psychosocial Well-Being." *The Lancet*, November 3.

Omidian, P. A. 2011. *When Bamboo Bloom: An Anthropologist in Taliban's Afghanistan.* Long Grove, IL: Waveland Press.

Omidian, P. A. 2012. "Developing Culturally Relevant Psychosocial Training for Afghan Teachers." *Intervention* 10(3): 237–248.

Omidian, P. A., and N. J. Lawrence. 2007. "A Community-Based Approach to Focusing: The Islam and Focusing Project of Afghanistan." *Folio: A Journal for Focusing and Experiential Therapy* 20(1): 152–162.

Omidian, P. A., and N. Papadopoulos. 2003. "Addressing Afghan Children's Psychosocial Needs in the Classroom: A Case Study of a Training for Trainers." IRC Female Education Program, Peshawar, Pakistan. Retrieved from http://healingclassrooms.org.

Orbinski, J. 2008. *An Imperfect Offering: Humanitarian Action for the Twenty-First Century*. New York: Walker & Co.

Panter-Brick, C. 2014. "Health, Risk, and Resilience: Interdisciplinary Concepts and Applications." *Annual Review of Anthropology* 43: 431–448.

Panter-Brick, C., and M. Eggerman. 2012. "Understanding Culture, Resilience, and Mental Health: The Production of Hope." In *The Social Ecology of Resilience: A Handbook of Theory and Practice*, edited by M. Ungar. New York: Springer, 369–386.

Pascale, R., J. Sternin, and M. Sternin. 2010. *The Power of Positive Deviance: How Unlikely Innovators Solve the World's Toughest Problems*. Boston, MA: Harvard Business Review Press.

Redfield, P. 2012. "The Unbearable Lightness of Ex-Pats: Double Bind of Humanitarian Mobility." *Cultural Anthropology* 27: 358–382.

Ud Din, I., Z. Mumtaz, and A. Ataullahjan. 2012. "How the Taliban Undermined Community Healthcare in Swat, Pakistan." *British Medical Journal* 344: e2093.

PART II

Iraq

5

War and the Public Health Disaster in Iraq

SCOTT HARDING AND KATHRYN LIBAL

Public health is directly shaped by war, conflict, and capitalism, yet exploring the connections between these processes remains neglected in scholarship and policymaking arenas. Such inquiry is vital to better understand how public health systems can be rebuilt following the cessation of violent conflict, which is critical to promoting individual well-being and supporting families and communities. Anthropologists have much to offer regarding the interconnections between health, war, and political economy. While the ethnography of war and political conflict are topics of lasting interest to anthropologists (Lubkemann 2008; Nordstrom 2004; Scheper-Hughes and Bourgois 2004), medical anthropology has not deeply examined the connections between war and health (Inhorn 2008). In her presidential address to the Society for Medical Anthropology in 2007, Marcia Inhorn signaled "chagrin over medical anthropology's relative apathy" (2008, 418) in the face of ongoing wars in the Middle East. She asserted:

> As a discipline, we have been faint of heart and lacking moral courage in this arena. In so doing, we have turned away from the brutal realities, the embodied suffering, the psychological devastation, the sexual violence, and the refugee aftermath of war. (421–422)

The history of Iraq illustrates that war is not an episodic and limited phenomenon; rather it is often a long-term, structural process with different phases, some more visible than others. Instead of a phenomenon that erupts by accident or as a result of historical enmity, war and other "complex emergencies" must be understood as intentional acts with their own politics, functions, and benefits (Keen 2008; Calhoun 2004). Thus, in most cases of war and other "man-made" disasters, global and local interests are profoundly intertwined. In chronic conflict—whether low intensity among local actors or high intensity involving local and international actors—key social institutions and the well-being of ordinary people are compromised in multiple ways. In particular, health outcomes diminish as the impacts of war become embedded in society over time. This is especially so in the case of Iraq, where powerful geopolitical actors such as the United States have sought to control local resources and populations.

Tracing the "costs" of war extends far beyond calculating the resources set aside for waging battle or keeping peace. War continues to have negative health consequences long after formal cessation of armed conflict. Aside from immediate destruction, war creates direct and indirect negative effects on health that can take generations to overcome (Inhorn 2008). War diverts resources to the military, fractures local community and creates forced displacement, undermines economic networks, and degrades the physical environment, thus jeopardizing food production and water quality. Violent conflict, by disrupting public health and other basic infrastructure, can create long-term conditions of famine and disease, often killing more people indirectly than who die from direct fighting (Krause and Mutimer 2005). This problem is acute in developing countries: Increased military spending in response to conflict typically continues after formal fighting ends, reducing spending on vital services like education and healthcare (Gupta et al. 2002). While the health effects of war are profound, they are often disregarded by powerful global actors and obscured by popular media accounts of most violent conflict.

The 2003 US invasion and the ongoing conflict in Iraq have destabilized an already fragile society and worsened social conditions for most people, while a public health disaster has silently unfolded.[1] The war has aggravated social divisions and fueled ethnic/sectarian conflict, fractured communities, undermined social development, and created a massive displaced population. Less noticed, stresses on the Iraqi healthcare system have increased since 2003, while the health and well-being of Iraqis have deteriorated.[2] High rates of mortality and morbidity related to the conflict, rising child and infant mortality, and the reliance of almost one-third of Iraqis on emergency aid all signal a deepening public health disaster (MedAct 2008).

The health crisis in Iraq must be understood in historical context, as Iraqis have experienced more than three decades of war and isolation from the international community. The Iran-Iraq War in the 1980s, the 1991 Gulf War, and more than a decade of UN-imposed economic sanctions contributed to the current humanitarian disaster. In particular, sanctions and a separate US trade embargo in the 1990s devastated social development, effectively dismantling Iraq's once impressive public health system (Garfield 1999; MedAct 2004; Popal 2000; Rawaf 2005). The current armed conflict in Iraq and its attendant effects have further undermined previous social progress and health gains. Moreover, US-backed neoliberal reconstruction policies implemented following the overthrow of Saddam Hussein have intensified these effects.

Since the 2003 invasion, US military operations, ethnic cleansing, and other targeted violence by Iraqis have intensified the scale of suffering and loss of life. Communities that had been ethnically and religiously diverse have been segregated into separate Shi'a and Sunni enclaves controlled by local militia, Iraqi security forces, or the US military. Because of this rising sectarianism, many Iraqis find it difficult to work, attend school, access healthcare, or obtain services. Despite a decline in violent deaths and large-scale attacks by 2008, human rights violations remain widespread, marked by indiscriminate killings, bombings, and kidnappings.

Although violence has increased in Iraq since the US invasion, Iraqis' well-being is also threatened by external factors. US-initiated neoliberal policies have helped foment the "sectarianization" of public services, including healthcare, and a continued degradation of key state functions. Hastily implemented privatization and the 2003 decision to "de-Baathify" the government and public sector undermined what weak health infrastructure remained after the sanctions era (Klein 2007; Phillips 2005). Because of ongoing violence and the fragmentation of the state, preventable disease, infant mortality, and "excess" deaths have increased in most of the country. Malnutrition, lack of sanitation and clean water, and limited access to medical services, resulting from pervasive conflict, contribute to these trends (MedAct 2008; UNICEF 2008a).

The ongoing crisis has also accelerated the dismantling of Iraq's medical system, as healthcare professionals have become the deliberate targets of insurgent groups as a weapon of war. With these providers increasingly at risk, Iraq faces a "brain drain" of the most qualified medical personnel, including the loss of educators training new doctors and nurses. In the long term this poses significant barriers to the reconstruction of the healthcare sector. In the short term, access to healthcare is uneven, with quality of care increasingly dependent on one's ability to pay for services. The limitation of "humanitarian space" for UN agencies or international NGOs to provide medical assistance compounds these challenges. Medecins Sans Frontieres and other health-related NGOs have resorted to using mobile clinics in Iraq, creating trauma units in neighboring countries, and training ordinary Iraqis in community health services to compensate for a degraded public health sector. Given the scale of displacement of Iraqis, the limited access to adequate primary healthcare and mental health services for some two million refugees living in Jordan, Syria, and other host countries represents another destructive effect of the war (Harper 2008; International Crisis Group 2008a; Libal and Harding 2009).

In short, the conflict in Iraq represents a compelling example of a "man-made disaster" (Harding 2007). Despite official statements of concern for Iraqis' well-being, humanitarian and health consequences of the war have been lesser concerns of US foreign policy than achieving geopolitical goals. We highlight the systemic effects on health of the US invasion of Iraq and chronic armed conflict that has ensued since 2003. We illustrate how the current conflict represents a continuation of external structural violence initiated in the 1990s in the form of economic sanctions and US foreign policy decisions. Under the rule of Saddam Hussein, and in the wake of his overthrow, internal and external policy decisions have slowly crippled state services, while social conditions in Iraq have deteriorated.[3]

The US Legacy: Political Instability and Violence

The 2003 US invasion of Iraq and overthrow of Saddam Hussein triggered massive internal destabilization in Iraq, which further undermined social development, health, and well-being in much of the country. The social fabric of local communities has been radically transformed, as many members of religious minority groups and families of mixed Shi'a and Sunni backgrounds have fled the country or have moved to "safer" neighborhoods and provinces. As a result of sectarian conflict, much of the central and southern provinces have been transformed into distinctly divided communities along ethnic and religious lines.

The ongoing US military occupation also complicates Iraq's political processes. By late 2008, there was little evidence of fundamental political reconciliation or progress on key policy issues (International Crisis Group 2008b). Despite US pressure to achieve a number of political "benchmarks," several of the most crucial initiatives have stalled. The existence of a civil war, failing state institutions, and deep ethnic, religious, and tribal cleavages thus compromise the future stability of Iraq and suggest that comprehensive social development via a strong government is a distant prospect. One analysis of weak and "failed states" ranked Iraq second worst in the world in terms of vulnerability to violent internal conflict and social dysfunction (Fund for Peace and Foreign Policy Magazine 2008).

The enactment of a "Baghdad Security Plan" and an increase ("surge") in US troops in 2007 appears to have helped reduce the level of violence and attacks on civilians and security forces. While more than 5,500 civilians died from violence in Baghdad province alone in the first quarter of 2007, according to government ministries (Susman 2007), by October the number of civilian deaths fell to approximately 1,000 a month (Buckley and Gordon 2007). The level of civilian casualties dropped by late 2008 to their lowest reported level since the war began (Brookings Institution 2008). This decrease reflects a combination of the end of the 2007 "surge," an agreement by followers of Moqtada al-Sadr to stop attacks against US forces, reduced armed violence among Shiite factions, and the incorporation of anti-US insurgents into "Awakening Councils" which focused on stabilizing local neighborhoods and targeting al Qaeda in Iraq (Galbraith 2008). Despite the apparent gains, violence against women, professional groups like academics, rising intolerance against minorities, and sectarian violence in those areas with diverse ethnic and religious groups remain especially problematic (UNAMI 2007a). Moreover, even though violence declined in late 2007, lawlessness remains endemic in central and southern Iraq.

Although levels of violence continued to drop throughout 2008, analysts suggest these gains could be quickly reversed and that instability continues to plague Iraq (Farrell and Oppel Jr. 2008; International Crisis

Group 2008b). The UN found that "continual fear from violence from all sides, including armed sectarian groups, criminal rackets, various militias, as well as during operations by security and military forces, is a daily reality for civilians" (UNAMI 2007c, 3). The International Committee of the Red Cross asserted that engaging in the mundane pursuits of everyday life—walking to school, shopping, riding the bus—were now matters of life and death (ICRC 2007). Fear of everyday violence in Iraq is particularly acute for women and girls, limiting their freedom of movement and ability to go to work or school (Susskind 2007).

Within this context, the rush to embrace lower levels of violence as proof of the "success" of US policy and the legitimacy of the Iraqi government is misleading. In reality, fundamental tensions among tribal, religious, and ethnic groups remain unresolved, while basic municipal services are an empty promise for most Iraqis. The central government remains weak, while heavily armed sectarian militias and insurgent groups bide their time as they consolidate control of different sectors of the government and economy. "Iraq still lacks the formal rules to divide the power and spoils of an oil-rich nation among ethnic, religious and tribal groups and unite them under one stable idea of Iraq. The improvements are fragile" (Farrell and Oppel 2008, A7). Overall, the political situation in Iraq remains divided on several key issues, including representation in national and provincial governments, proposed legislation related to oil revenue sharing, and the status of Kirkuk.

The Politics of Denial: The Death Toll in Iraq

US forces in Iraq have never provided data on civilian casualties and deaths. Distancing themselves from "body counts" of the Vietnam War, the Bush administration claimed that counting civilian casualties was not a part of the US mission. While the Iraqi government attempted to count bodies processed through morgues, it ended this practice reportedly under pressure from the US and Iraqi governments (Steele and Goldenberg 2008).

Several organizations and scholars have attempted to estimate Iraqi deaths using different methodologies (Roberts et al. 2004). Their estimates of civilian deaths vary widely, and each has generated controversy. The UN, using information from the Iraqi government, hospitals, and healthcare officials, reported that 34,352 civilians died in violence in 2006 alone (UNAMI 2007a). The Iraqi government claimed some 150,000 civilians had been killed between 2004 and 2006 (Oppel Jr. 2006). The Iraq Body Count, an independent public database of violent civilian deaths derived from media reports in Iraq resulting from the 2003 US military intervention, suggested a death toll (as of April 2009) of approximately 91,000–100,000 (Iraq Body Count 2009). Other research found an ("excess") civilian death toll from 2003 to 2006 of approximately 600,000 (Burnham et al. 2006). The latter estimates, published in *The Lancet*, were based on the second Iraqi household survey conducted by researchers at Johns Hopkins University. At the time, this represented a civilian casualty figure of approximately 2.5 percent of Iraq's population, dramatically higher than any other study had found. Somewhat predictably, this publication generated controversy over the findings and methodology used. Both surveys were dismissed by the US and British governments and criticized by some researchers (Daponte 2007; Hicks 2006); it received minimal media coverage, especially in the United States (Tirman 2008).

In early 2008, the World Health Organization (WHO) estimated that 151,000 violent deaths occurred from March 2003 through June 2006 (Iraq Family Health Survey Study Group 2008). This was more than triple the Iraq Body Count estimates for the same period. The WHO survey, based on a household survey with 9,345 heads of households, found that "violence is a leading cause of death for Iraqi adults and was the main cause of death in men between the ages of 15 and 59 years during the first 3 years after the 2003 invasion" (484).

A much higher casualty figure was produced by a prominent British polling firm in January 2008. The group estimated "that over 1,000,000 Iraqi citizens have died as a result of the conflict which started in 2003" (Opinion Research Business 2008). This meant that some 20 percent of Iraqis had experienced at least one death in their household due to the ongoing conflict rather than from natural causes. According to the report, in August 2007 the group found that 1.2 million Iraqis had died since 2003, and they decided to conduct additional research in rural areas of Iraq to enhance the validity of their research. These findings generated scant attention in the US media or among organizations addressing the Iraq conflict (Tirman 2008).

Although data on violent civilian deaths vary widely, even the lowest estimates reveal a dramatic level of violence in Iraq since 2003. As troubling has been the relative silence by the international community and US media about the loss of life in Iraq. Similarly, little notice has been paid to the changing life expectancy rates in Iraq. The life expectancy rate at birth in 2008 was 57 years (WHO 2008). Life expectancy in Iraq had dramatically improved in the late 1970s and 1980s, and then began to decline with the onset of economic sanctions and the violence surrounding the US invasion. WHO data rank Iraq 119th in the world in life expectancy in data published in 2018.

The Human Costs of Economic Sanctions and War in Iraq

When considering the dismantling of modern Iraqi society, an historical perspective that includes an assessment of external influences on state capacity illustrates the civilian consequences of war and militarism. The Iran-Iraq War (1980–1988) devastated Iraq's economy and undermined gains in living standards, yet by 1990 Iraq still ranked second highest in human development in the Middle East (Pedersen 2007). Thus, the damage inflicted by the US military in the first Gulf War and from UN sanctions (1990–2003), along with the ongoing conflict, bears much responsibility for the shift from an increasingly self-sufficient country to a failed state.

The state of health, nutrition, and well-being under sanctions contrasts with Iraq's relatively affluent status in 1990. Before the 1991 Gulf War, Iraq invested heavily in the health sector, making primary medical care available to most urban residents and some 80 percent of the rural population. Infant and child mortality had been reduced significantly during the 1980s, while water and sanitation treatment services "were well developed" (UNICEF 1998, 7). Until the mid-1980s, in terms of social development Iraq was "fast approaching standards comparable to those of developed countries" (UNDP 2002, 11). This perspective was echoed by a European doctor we interviewed, who was involved in humanitarian relief in Iraq during the First Gulf War and participated in international planning teams for health reconstruction following the 2003 invasion. He asserted that Iraq's achievements in primary health had been significant; Iraq had better vaccination rates and was outperforming many European countries.

Much of Iraq's infrastructure was destroyed by US bombing in the Gulf War. This damage, combined with the onset of sanctions, precipitated a public health crisis, as malnutrition and the rate of water-borne diseases erupted in 1991 (Hiltermann 1991; Ascherio et al. 1992). Sanctions undermined the ability of the public health system and social infrastructure to address healthcare and nutrition. Iraq's healthcare system, formerly among the most developed in the region, was seriously degraded (Popal 2000). By the time of the 2003 US invasion, "the public health system was in tatters, it was under-resourced, and the population was economically deprived," noted an interviewee. As Iraq's economy withered, child malnutrition, disease, and infant and child mortality increased sharply in the 1990s, and food self-sufficiency declined (Dobson 2000; Garfield 1999; UNICEF 1998). Sanctions were chiefly responsible for the excess deaths of 300,000–500,000 infants and children during the 1990s (Garfield and Leu 2000). By 2003 the UN found that more than one-fifth of Iraq's population in its most populated areas was "chronically poor" and nearly two-thirds of Iraqis were dependent on government food rations (UN World Food Programme 2003). Thus, under sanctions Iraq "experienced a shift from relative affluence to massive poverty" (UNDP 2002, 12).

While obtaining current figures on social indicators is difficult, available data suggest that the overall health of much of the Iraqi population is precarious (MedAct 2008; UNICEF 2008b; UNHCR 2008). Despite some economic and social progress since 2003, the US-led war has created a deepening disaster for Iraqis in terms of social development and public health. A comprehensive household survey in 2004 found deteriorating physical and social conditions. Electrical, water, and sewer systems were deeply compromised and unreliable, further endangering health. Since that study, conditions have declined significantly. More than half of Iraqis live on less than $1 a day, unemployment ranges from 25 to 40 percent, and more than eight million people are categorized as "poor" (UNAMI 2007b, 2007c).

A lack of medicines, equipment, and healthcare personnel has imperiled an already fragile health service system. UNICEF reported that the ongoing conflict and under-investment in infrastructure have "undermined Iraq's vital social services to the point where many basic family needs are going unmet" (UNICEF 2008a). The UNICEF Special

Representative for Iraq found that a lack of hygiene and safe drinking water are "priority concerns for Iraqi families" and young children are particularly affected by waterborne diseases and malnutrition. IOM reported that "water and sewage systems in the country are generally poorly functioning and dilapidated. In places where water networks/sewage systems exist or connect to areas they are either overstretched . . . or deficient" (IOM 2008a, 14). Reflecting the degraded water and sanitation systems, a cholera outbreak occurred in late 2007 in Baghdad and parts of Kurdish Iraq (UNAMI 2007c).

Costs for basic (and private) healthcare in Iraq have also risen, drugs and other critical supplies are often non-existent, and there exists an acute shortage of hospital beds. Most hospitals and primary healthcare centers in the southern and central Governorates are operating in substandard condition. As one UN official in an interview with us noted,

> A lot of the health facilities do not have medications they need. They are overstretched—there are too many people going there and they don't have the simple equipment. Sometimes the equipment is broken down and can't be replaced or it is stolen during the earlier part of the war. So the health conditions are very, very poor.

Thus, as the International Committee for the Red Cross underscores, "five years after the war began, many Iraqis do not have access to the most basic health care . . . The Iraqi health-care system is now in worse shape than ever. Many lives have been lost because prompt and appropriate medical care is not available" (ICRC 2008, 8).

Food security is precarious for Iraqis in central and southern Governorates. In 2003, the World Food Programme conducted a food security assessment and found that some 11 percent (2.6 million people) were "extremely poor and vulnerable to food insecurity" (UNWFP/COSIT 2006, 1). At that time, if the PDS program was eliminated, another 3.6 million Iraqis would be food insecure. In a follow-up survey in 2006, the WFP found that 15 percent of Iraqis (some 4 million people) were food insecure and "in dire need of different types of humanitarian assistance, including food," despite receiving public food rations (2). The survey also found that "a further 8.3 million people (31.8 percent of the surveyed population) would be rendered food insecure if they were not provided with a PDS ration."

Hunger and malnutrition have a devastating effect on children; between 1990 and 2005, the increase in infant mortality in Iraq (150 percent) was the highest in the world (Save the Children 2007). An estimated 19 percent of Iraqi children suffered from malnutrition under sanctions, while 28 percent were malnourished by 2007 (NGO Coordination Committee in Iraq and Oxfam 2007, 3). Child mortality rates, which soared in the 1990s, have worsened since 2003. Only 30 percent of Iraqi children are estimated to have access to clean water (UNICEF 2007). One in eight Iraqi children died in 2005 before their fifth birthday; more than half of these deaths occurred among babies younger than one month old (Save the Children 2007). Declining school enrollment also reveals the disintegration of social institutions that assure children's well-being. The Iraqi Ministry of Education reported that 30 percent of elementary school children attended school in 2007, a sharp decline from figures of 75 percent in 2006 (Amnesty International 2008).

Particularly detrimental to the long-term stability of Iraq is the mental health impact of pervasive violence and family and community disintegration, especially on children (UNICEF 2007; MedAct 2004). While surveys of children's mental health and the effects of the war have been limited, the World Health Organization found that in areas hard hit by violence up to 30 percent of Iraqi children suffer from a posttraumatic stress disorder (UNICEF 2007). With mental health services already scarce before the 2003 US invasion, those suffering trauma as a result of the current conflict have few viable treatment options (Al-Jadiry and Rustam 2006; Curie 2006). A recent study found that a lack of community support and pervasive stigma toward those with mental illness prevented 65 percent of patients in Iraq's only long-term mental health facility from family and community reintegration (Humaidi 2006). The significance of the gap in mental health services cannot be understated: Political and social reconciliation must be seen as linked to the ability to deal with the long-term effects of such trauma on a generation of Iraqis.

The disintegration of key social institutions (especially in the central and southern provinces) and endemic conflict in Baghdad and other cities have forced large numbers of Iraqis to leave their homes. The UN estimates some 2.2 million refugees have fled to neighboring countries, while 2.8 million Iraqis are considered "internally displaced persons," or IDPs (IOM 2008a). According to aid workers we interviewed, Iraqi refugees are among the most traumatized that they have encountered in recent decades. A recent study of Jordan and Lebanon found that a high percentage of Iraqi families are "undergoing a period of serious emotional and psychosocial threats. These threats create widespread distress in (the) living environment of displaced Iraqis" (IOM 2008b, 14). Refugees in Syria reported "a high exposure to distressing and traumatic events" in Iraq, such as being a victim of violence, kidnappings, and torture, as well as displacement itself. Related to this, "high incidences of domestic violence as well as anxiety and depression" have been reported among Iraqi refugees in Syria (ICMC 2008, 8). Yet, as in Iraq, mental health services for refugees are severely limited in Jordan and Syria, where the majority of Iraqi refugees reside.

Few systematic studies have been done on the mental health needs of displaced Iraqis. A 2004 survey of refugees living in London found high levels of distress and mental health needs, concluding that in general, "a high proportion of Iraqi refugee family members constitute a population at risk for adjustment and mental health problems" (Hosin, Moore, and Gaitanou 2006, 129). Given that this research predates the period when violence in Iraq escalated, the mental health needs of more recent Iraqi refugees is likely even more profound.

Though refugees have garnered more media attention since 2007, IDPs in Iraq are increasingly vulnerable and lack critical protections, and their material conditions are less well documented. The UN found that many internally displaced Iraqis cannot access needed medicines, adequate housing, or work (UNAMI 2007c). In one-third of Iraq's eighteen Governorates, more than 25 percent of IDPs lack regular access to water (IOM 2008a). Some relief workers worry that those Iraqis who are too poor to move at all remain the most vulnerable, for they lack the networks and resources to move to safer and better functioning communities. As one UN official working with IDPs told us in an interview in July 2008:

> There are just many, many reasons why being displaced is not an ideal situation . . . [T]he choice is you and your family members get killed or

you leave. . . . But increasingly the conditions for the displaced are deteriorating and I think many Iraqis are realizing that leaving is just not a very good option [either].

The "Brain Drain" and Its Consequences on Healthcare

While the flow of refugees from Iraq has garnered notice, little attention has been paid to *who* exactly has left the country and its implication for long-term stability and the redevelopment of Iraq. A discernable "brain drain" has emerged, as academics and intellectuals, trained medical professionals, former government workers, entrepreneurs, the middle class, and the wealthy have fled the violence and persecution engulfing much of Iraq (Sassoon 2009; UNAMI 2007a).

The ability of key state institutions to function effectively is threatened by the loss of skilled workers, trained specialists, and administrators. As of late 2007, an estimated 40 percent of professionals have fled Iraq since 2003 (Brookings Institution 2007). Key sectors of Iraqi society have been disproportionately affected. For example, more than half of Iraq's registered physicians are estimated to have left the country (ICRC 2008; MedAct 2008). Trained specialists, the backbone of Iraq's healthcare system, are increasingly in short supply as most have also fled violence and persecution. The head of the Iraqi Doctors' Syndicate estimated that between 60 and 70 percent of physicians with 15–20 years' experience have left Iraq, and an even higher percentage of those with more experience have fled (Kami 2008).

Another way the ongoing crisis has accelerated the dismantling of Iraq's medical system is that healthcare professionals have become the deliberate targets of violence as a "weapon of war" by assassinations or threats of violence against them or family members. Physicians have been a particular object of violence, while thousands of other healthcare workers have been subject to kidnapping, violence, and intimidation, helping to fuel this flight of trained medical specialists (Brookings Institution 2007; ICRC 2008; MedAct 2008; UNAMI 2007b). An estimated 2,000 Iraqi physicians have been murdered since the 2003 US invasion, with hundreds more kidnapped (Brookings Institution 2008). In an interview, a UN official noted that even monitoring health conditions in Iraq has become dangerous for their Iraqi workers. A humanitarian representative underscored that the health professionals they collaborated with in Iraq were at great risk: "Hospitals are targets; patients coming into hospitals are targets; patients inside hospitals are targets." In this climate, "everybody is afraid of everybody."

Interviews with humanitarian NGOs underscore that skilled medical personnel are now in short supply in Iraq, while access to adequate healthcare is inconsistent, especially for those with conflict-related injuries or chronic health conditions. One respondent in our study asserted that any doctor who could leave had already done so: "Everybody's left . . . [We have] got a country which was functioning in pre '91 on a European level—let's say Kuwait in the Middle East. [Now] we've gone to an Afghanistan level." The return of medical professionals following reconciliation between factions will be essential to the revival of healthcare in Iraq as will the training of a new generation of physicians and other health professionals.

Teachers and academics have also been persecuted, as Iraq's education sector has been similarly undermined. According to MedAct, the current crisis has created a "poorly trained, overworked, demoralized, fearful, underpaid health workforce" (2008, 5). While this development has been neglected in US debates about the Iraq war, the short- and long-term impact on health seems clear: "Iraqis describe their health system as 'beheaded,' because many of its brightest and best have already migrated, while the practitioners, managers, and teachers of the future are not being developed or supported" (ibid.).

While some professionals fled beginning in the 1970s, the current refugee flow suggests the creation of a new Iraqi diaspora. This development highlights the barriers to return migration of Iraqi refugees and the impact on long-term reconstruction efforts. Many of those fleeing Iraq today represent the best hopes for the creation of a vibrant, nonsectarian civil society and strong government. Based on a recent survey of Iraqi refugees (UNHCR 2008), as well as historical examples of other civil wars and refugee flows, it is unlikely that most Iraqi refugees will return without a drastic shift in the political and security environment. This assessment was shared with us by NGO and UN representatives working with Iraqi refugees in Jordan and Syria.

Although the likelihood of migration by professionals differs by occupation, the negative impact on key social institutions like healthcare is significant (Chikanda 2006). Thus, the ability to rebuild the Iraqi healthcare system faces a number of challenges. A culture of medical migration to the west already exists in other developing countries, with many physicians and skilled health personnel fleeing conflict and political violence (Hagopian et al. 2005). Without addressing militarism and fundamental political conflict, Iraq risks falling prey to similar institutional factors that have undermined public health elsewhere in the developing world.

In the interim, the larger political disputes dividing Iraq are evidenced in the structure and governance of the current health system. Healthcare provision and policy planning are managed through the patchwork efforts of the Ministry of Health, UN organizations, and international NGOs. A weak, fractured government has been unable to overcome its differences and promote development that addresses the decline in public health. Indeed, in many respects political and military conflict in Iraq has fueled the division of key services and government ministries among competing and sectarian groups (Marfleet 2007). The Ministry of Health has struggled to shed an image of representing sectarian Shi'a interests, while maintaining leadership that can implement a coherent health agenda. Perceived sectarianism has had a profound impact on access to healthcare. As one aid worker put it, "You want the doctor because he is a good doctor, you don't want him because he's Shi'a or Muslim or Sunni Muslim or Communist or Kurd." Turnover has been particularly high in administrative positions within the Ministry of Health and in hospitals in areas with high levels of armed conflict. Two informants noted that while in 2008 the upper leadership of the Ministry of Health stabilized, prior to that, high staff turnover resulted in incoherent policy and allowed privatization of health to occur. UN and independent analysts are troubled by trends related to the deregulation of the health sector and the long-term consequences this poses for ordinary Iraqis:

> The unregulated health economy, the need to maximize professional income, and the individualistic, specialty-focused traditions of Iraqi medicine are creating a fragmented fee-for-service system mainly delivering curative care. This cannot meet basic health needs effectively, and is beyond the average citizen's pocket. (MedAct 2008, 2)

"Disaster Capitalism": The Privatization of Health Reconstruction

The entangled relationship of war-making and capitalism has recently come under scrutiny (Klein 2007; Mattei and Nader 2008). The assimilation of national and local economies within a global system has profound consequences for developing societies. When the imperative to "integrate" is mandated by external actors, neoliberal policies can become catalysts for the intensification of violence. The harmful consequences of structural adjustment programs on the public sector in developing countries have been well documented (Kim et al. 2002). Badawi (2004) argues that globalization is most dangerous when developing countries are forced "to adopt certain structural and economic changes, which prematurely decrease expenditures on social services, including healthcare" (76). This challenge is amplified in countries where the state is weak and challenged by internal conflict, occupation, or war, such as in contemporary Iraq (Docena 2007).

Given the sophisticated state of Iraq's healthcare into the 1980s, the decline of its health infrastructure and Iraqis' well-being is all the more dramatic. While some have blamed current health failures on the rule of Saddam Hussein, regime change and the introduction of neoliberal economic policies bear a special responsibility for the health crisis. Shortly after the United States invaded Iraq in 2003, Paul Bremer, administrator of the Coalition Provisional Authority, enacted several transitional laws that undermined the already weak healthcare sector. His first major reform, Order #1, was to fire some 500,000 state workers, including soldiers, professors, teachers, doctors, nurses, engineers, and judges (Klein 2007). This policy became known as "de-Baathification." Bremer's program to "de-Baathify" the government extended too deeply into the public sector to be considered merely an effort to purge Hussein loyalists. Instead, Bremer sought to radically "downsize" the public sector, adhering to neoliberal principles of privatizing government-run industries, eliminating subsidies, and firing state workers (Docena 2007).

The ideological fixation with privatizing the Iraqi state is apparent in numerous accounts of "postwar" US policies. David L. Phillips, a former senior advisor to the State Department, finds that de-Baathification "was about distributing power to Iraqis who subscribed to the vision of the new Iraq" (Phillips 2005, 146). The Bush administration, in part, framed the invasion of Iraq as an opportunity to spread democracy in the Middle East. In practice this vision meant implementing a neoliberal agenda by purging those who opposed economic liberalization.

The neoliberals "believed that privatization would open Iraq to foreign investment, bring in foreign companies, and create an Iraqi bourgeoisie whose prosperity would inspire Syrians, Iranians, and others to seek the same" (Phillips 2005, 147). Indeed, through a series of orders issued by Bremer from May 2003 to June 2004, the United States instituted radical reforms to transform Iraq. Based on a plan written by the multinational corporation BearingPoint Inc. (formerly KPMG Consulting), these orders devolved public services and privatized key economic functions formerly performed by Iraq (Juhasz 2007).

Privatization and de-Baathification have entailed a reconstruction process characterized by systemic cost overruns, failure to prioritize healthcare and other human services, inability to complete projects, and corruption. As a result, transnational corporations have been enriched at the expense of Iraqis and US taxpayers. While US-funded programs have garnered attention, the limited spending on healthcare illustrates how public services fare poorly when militarism takes precedence. The Special Inspector General for Iraq Reconstruction (SIGIR) has provided insight into the challenges of reconstruction initiated during the Iraq War. SIGIR was highly critical of two contracts for healthcare infrastructure. An April 2006 audit of a $243 million contract with Parsons Delaware Inc. revealed that after almost $186 million had been spent over two years, only six primary healthcare centers were completed and 135 of 150 planned centers were partially constructed (SIGIR 2008). Of the latter, 121 centers were later "terminated for convenience." According to SIGIR, the contractor and US Agency for International Development (USAID) were responsible for the failure to complete the health centers.

SIGIR's 2006 audit of Bechtel's contract to build the Basra Children's Hospital found that an original estimate of $50 million in construction costs ballooned to a projected $150 million. Again, the Inspector General cited USAID management failures, noting that only three USAID officers were overseeing $1.4 billion in contracts. Thus, while the United States has modestly invested in new healthcare facilities, such efforts have been marred by delays, cost overruns, poor quality, a failure to address the long-term consequences of sanctions, and the impact of looting and deterioration since 2003.

Privatization also extends to humanitarian relief efforts. US-funded NGO work in Iraq is concentrated among a few players, including International Medical Corps, CARE, and Mercy Corps, and a number of for-profits. Breaking from past practices of funding UN agencies, these health-related contracts were disproportionately awarded to the private sector. Yet several agencies and corporations engaged in technical assistance and development projects have been criticized for failing to work effectively with Iraqis in developing health policy and programs.

Conclusion: Challenges to Creating Health Policy and Reconstruction of the Health Sector

US policies to invade Iraq, de-Baathify the government, and implement neoliberal economic policies represent one facet of the structural violence Iraqis have faced since 2003. Coupled with the long-term degradation of health infrastructure, the flight of healthcare professionals, and ongoing political conflict, Iraq requires full engagement of the international community to resolve its multiple and intertwined social, governance, and health crises.

Addressing the chronic material deprivation and multiple forms of mental health stress experienced by vulnerable Iraqis will require investment in health and educational policies that are comprehensive and sustained. Without a commitment to public health intervention, Iraq faces a future marred by the effects of declining health, pervasive trauma, and social exclusion. This latter condition is profound for youth and the elderly. Such problems will require substantial attention, yet adequate psychosocial supports are lacking in Iraq, within neighboring states hosting most Iraqi refugees, and to a lesser extent in western states that have resettled Iraqi refugees. An added complication are the cultural barriers among Iraqis to seeking professional mental health services due to the stigma attached to psychosocial problems (ICMC 2008). These limitations are also pronounced for the sizeable community of Iraqis with physical disabilities. In an interview, a caseworker specializing in disabilities with experience in the Middle East noted that thirty years of conflict in Iraq has created a disability crisis. She described a situation where a large number of Iraqis with physical disabilities are confined to their homes and lack services and community support. The current war has amplified their social isolation.

Given the fractured state of the health sector, NGOs have played important roles in providing technical assistance and healthcare services to Iraqis in recent years. This reflects, in part, the UN's absence from Iraq due to security concerns and political instability. Yet international NGOs that operate alongside Iraqi counterparts are forced to maintain a low profile because of the targeting of humanitarian actors. Thus, it remains difficult to comprehensively assess the impact of their efforts related to health and other unmet needs, while the effects of US reconstruction on public health have been decidedly mixed.

Inhorn's (2008) admonishment of anthropologists to research the effects of war on health, particularly in Iraq and Afghanistan, demands a response. In Iraq, the work to uncover how US military power and neoliberal reconstruction programs have contributed to the degradation of the public health system and health and well-being of Iraqis will require sustained and innovative research. It is vital that such analysis flourish in coming years in order to create momentum within the international community to address Iraq's public health crisis. Doing so will help ensure the rebuilding of Iraq's public health system and other key institutions and that those responsible for violations of human rights are held accountable.

Postscript

The case of Iraq demonstrates the relevance of understanding the "syndemics of war" (Ostrach and Singer 2013). Numerous examples in this chapter indicate that the effects of armed conflict cause long-term disruption to healthcare systems and social infrastructure, which in turn undermines community functioning and individual health and well-being. The 2003 invasion and occupation of Iraq by external actors, such as the United States, created a cascade of adverse social and political consequences, exacerbating existing chronic negative trends. Despite the formal end of US combat operations in Iraq in 2010, stability, reconstruction, and peace have not materialized. Iraqis' social and economic vulnerability is exacerbated by the political failures of the government and external actors, such as the United States. Open conflict continues in central and northern Iraq and new forms of sectarian authoritarianism, repression, and state corruption have emerged as social forces that continue to threaten stability (Sassoon 2016).

Critical infrastructure, such as health facilities, educational institutions, sanitation, and water systems, has not been restored to prewar standards. The recent UK-commissioned "Report of the Iraq Inquiry" notes that the British (and by extension US) government failed to adequately consider the "likely and actual effects" of military action that were bound to entail "not only direct civilian casualties, but also the indirect costs on civilians arising from worsening social, economic, and health conditions" (as cited in Webster 2016, 226). Webster details the continuing deterioration of the Iraqi healthcare system due to "severe budgetary shortfalls created by low oil prices, and the displacement of millions of civilians due to conflict between government troops and insurgents" as well as "deep corruption within Iraq's health-care system" (ibid.). Thus, we must regard such "social facts" as persistent child malnutrition/stunting and high rates of neonatal deaths as a consequence of decades of war-making in Iraq. And, illustrative of Ostrach and Singer's (2013) "syndemics of war," these harmful conditions are in turn tied to food insecurity, lack of access to safe water, and weak healthcare infrastructure. In sum, Iraq exemplifies Ostrach and Singer's assertion that "war is a traumatic and disruptive biosocial process that sets in motion dynamic interactions between diseases and other health conditions that significantly increase war-related morbidity and mortality" (258).

These consequences have persisted, despite the end of major US military involvement, as Iraq has continued to experience the effects of geopolitical conflict. For example, the war in Syria and the subsequent rise of the Islamic State of Iraq and Syria (ISIS) has triggered a new conflict with predictable results on Iraqi society. By capturing territory in Syria and northern Iraq, including Mosul, and establishing a self-proclaimed caliphate, ISIS exacerbated ethnic and religious tensions (Human Rights Watch 2018). The targeting of minority groups, such as the Yazidi, created a new wave of internal displacement; while many of the estimated one million Iraqi refugees who resided in Syria were forced to return to Iraq or seek refuge in another country (Cetorelli, Burnham, and Shabila

2017). In response, the Iraqi military, supported by the United States, launched renewed large-scale military operations in northern Iraq in an effort to defeat ISIS.

Thus, while the US military presence waned, armed conflict and direct violence has remained a reality for Iraqis. Accurately measuring the costs, however, has proven challenging (Levy and Sidel 2013). One estimate of direct civilian deaths caused by violence in Iraq since the 2003 US invasion finds that approximately 200,000 Iraqis have been killed. That figure rises to nearly 300,000 violent deaths when armed combatants are included (Iraq Body Count 2018). These are conservative figures, based only on recorded, direct violent (civilian) deaths, and they do not include deaths stemming from displacement, damage to infrastructure, disease, and/or lack of access to healthcare, clean water, and food. Other research supports a significantly higher death toll among civilians (as suggested in this chapter). Physicians for Social Responsibility (2015) thus found that, "directly or indirectly . . . around 1 million people in Iraq" died as a result of war, occupation, and indirect effects. That estimate came before a new wave of violence linked to ISIS and the effort to defeat them.

Iraq declared victory against ISIS in late 2017. Yet the degraded state of Iraq's healthcare system and infrastructure, and its weakened economy, implies that many more *indirect* deaths will occur in future years. The failure to resolve Iraq's myriad political conflicts suggests that the potential for renewed fighting is likely and political fragmentation and corruption remain daunting challenges, leaving the people in Iraq in a vulnerable state. The deterioration of major social institutions, such as education and health systems, and more than two decades of forced migration of Iraqis to other countries—hallmarks of war—impede Iraq's stabilization and recovery to pre-1990s levels.

NOTES

1 The term "Iraqi" is a political construct that some communities in Iraq may not recognize, in particular, Kurds who seek an independent state. We use this term because it is the dominant frame of reference for most academic, official, and journalistic discourse.
2 Given the lack of reliable research that disaggregates health data on the basis of region, ethnic or religious group affiliation, it is difficult to generalize about the well-being of Kurds versus Shi'a or Sunni Arabs in Iraq. Much data collection

in Iraq on health and other social indicators over the past two decades has been rudimentary. In spite of these constraints there is a growing body of data gathered in surveys collected by UN agencies, the government of Iraq, and different nongovernmental organizations. Future research must better address differences in health infrastructure and outcomes by region, social class, and ethnic and religious affiliation.

3 Our chapter is part of a larger study on NGO advocacy for displaced Iraqis that we began in late 2006. We conducted interviews and fieldwork in Jordan, Syria, Turkey, and the United States, with more than 60 respondents working in humanitarian and human rights NGOs, the US Congress, and UN agencies. We have not done interviews in Iraq, reflecting our reluctance to enter field sites in which both researchers and informants are vulnerable. In the United States, we interviewed NGO representatives engaged in advocacy and direct service to Iraqi refugees, and staff from Congress and the State Department. In 2007 and 2008 we spent two months in Jordan, Syria, and Turkey, interviewing informants from international and local NGOs, specifically those who are or have been providing assistance to Iraqi refugees in Jordan, and the United Nations. We also interviewed several key respondents who played important roles in assessing and creating health policy in Iraq as well as UN officials. We did semi-structured interviews, with an emphasis on understanding the politics of NGO advocacy and the provision of humanitarian assistance. We asked informants about the social costs of endemic conflict in Iraq, the specific needs of Iraqi refugees, barriers to healthcare and service provision, the capacity of local and international NGOs to provide services, the role of key global actors like the United States and UN, and the various strategy and tactics of advocacy on this issue by NGOs.

REFERENCES

Al-Jadiry, Abdul-Monaf, and Hussain Rustam. 2006. "Mental Health Education and Training in Iraq: An Overview." *Journal of Muslim Mental Health* 1, no. 2: 117–122.

Amnesty International. 2008. *Carnage and Despair in Iraq: Iraq Five Years On*. London: Amnesty International.

Ascherio, Albert, Robert Chase, Tim Cote, Godelieave Dehaes, Eric Hoskins, Jilali Laaouej, Megan Passey, Saleh Qaderi, Saher Shuqaidef, Mary C. Smith, et al. 1992. "Effect of the Gulf War on Infant and Child Mortality in Iraq." *New England Journal of Medicine* 327, no. 13: 931–936.

Badawi, Aboubakr A. 2004. "The Social Dimension of Globalization and Health." *Perspectives on Global Development and Technology* 3, no. 1–2: 73–90.

Brookings Institution. 2007. *The Iraq Index. Tracking Variables of Reconstruction and Security in Post-Saddam Iraq*, November 29. Washington, DC.

———. 2008. *The Iraq Index. Tracking Variables of Reconstruction and Security in Post-Saddam Iraq*, November 6. Washington, DC.

Buckley, Cara, and Michael R. Gordon. 2007, November 19. "U.S. Says Attacks in Iraq Fell to the Level of February 2006." *New York Times*, A1, A6.

Burnham, Gilbert, Riyadh Lafta, Shannon Doocy, and Les Roberts. 2006. "Mortality after the 2003 Invasion of Iraq: A Cross-Sectional Cluster Sample Survey." *The Lancet* 368, no. 9545: 1421–1428.

Calhoun, Craig. 2004. "A World of Emergencies: Fear, Intervention, and the Limits of Cosmopolitan Order." *Canadian Review of Sociology and Anthropology* 41, no. 4: 373–395.

Cetorelli, Valeria, Gilbert Burnham, and Nazar Shabila. 2017. "Health Needs and Health Care Seeking Behaviors of Yazidis and Other Minority Groups Displaced by ISIS into the Kurdistan Region of Iraq." *PLoS ONE* 12, 8, 1–10. doi.org/10.1371/journal.pone.0181028.

Chikanda, Abel. 2006. "Skilled Health Professionals' Migration and Its Impact on Health Delivery in Zimbabwe. *Journal of Ethnic and Migration Studies* 32, no. 4: 667–680.

Curie, Charles G. 2006. "Health Diplomacy in Action: Helping Iraq Rebuild Its Mental Health System." *Journal of Muslim Mental Health* 1, no. 2: 109–116.

Daponte, Beth O. 2007. "Wartime Estimates of Iraqi Civilian Casualties." *International Review of the Red Cross* 89, no. 868: 943–957.

Dobson, Roger. 2000. "Sanctions against Iraq 'Double' Child Mortality." *British Medical Journal* 321, no. 7275: 1490.

Docena, Herbert. 2007. "Free Market by Force: The Making and Un-making of a Neo-liberal Iraq." *International Journal of Contemporary Iraqi Studies* 1, no. 2: 123–142.

Farrell, S., and R. A. Oppel, Jr. 2008, June 21. "Big Gains for Iraq Security, but Questions Linger." *New York Times*, A1, A7.

Fund for Peace and Foreign Policy Magazine. 2008. *The Failed States Index*, July/August. Retrieved from http://www.foreignpolicy.com.

Galbraith, Peter W. 2008. "Is This a 'Victory'?" *New York Review of Books* 55, October 15, no. 16.

Garfield, Richard. 1999. *The Impact of Economic Sanctions on Health and Well-Being*. Relief and Rehabilitation Network, Overseas Development Institute.

Garfield, Richard, and C. S. Leu. 2000. "A Multivariate Method for Estimating Mortality Rates among Children under 5 Years from Health and Social Indicators in Iraq." *International Journal of Epidemiology* 29: 510–515.

Gupta, Sanjeev, Benedict Clements, Rina Bhattacharya, and Shamit Chakravarti. 2002. "The Elusive Peace Dividend." *Finance and Development* 39, no. 4: 49–51.

Hagopian, Amy, Anthony Ofosu, Adesegun Fatusi, Richard Biritwum, Ama Essel, L. Gary Hart, and Carolyn Watts. 2005. "The Flight of Physicians from West Africa: Views of African Physicians and Implications for Policy." *Social Science and Medicine* 61: 1750–1760.

Harding, Scott. 2007. "Man-made Disaster and Development: The Case of Iraq." *International Social Work* 50, no. 3: 295–306.

Harper, Andrew. 2008. "Iraq's Refugees: Ignored and Unwanted." *International Review of the Red Cross* 90, no. 869: 169–190.

Hicks, Madelyn H. 2006. *Mortality after the 2003 Invasion of Iraq: Were Valid and Ethical Field Methods Used in This Survey?* Households in Conflict Network Research Design Note 3. Institute of Development Studies, University of Essex.

Hiltermann, Joost R. 1991. "Assessing the Damage in Iraq." *Journal of Palestine Studies* 20, no. 4: 109–114.

Hosin, Amer A., Simon Moore, and Christina Gaitanou. 2006. "The Relationship between Psychological Well-Being and Adjustment of Both Parents and Children of Exiled and Traumatized Iraqi Refugees." *Journal of Muslim Mental Health* 1, no. 2: 123–136.

Humaidi, Naama S. 2006. "Resettlement Prospects for Inpatients at Al Rashad Mental Hospital." *Journal of Muslim Mental Health* 1, no, 2: 177–183.

Human Rights Watch. 2018. "Iraq: Events of 2017." In *Human Rights Watch World Report 2018*. Retrieved from www.hrw.org.

Inhorn, Marcia C. 2008. "Medical Anthropology against War." *Medical Anthropology Quarterly* 22, no. 4: 416–424.

International Catholic Migration Commission (ICMC). 2008. *Iraqi Refugees in Syria*. Washington, DC: ICMC.

International Committee of the Red Cross (ICRC). 2007. *Iraq: Civilians Without Protection. The Ever-worsening Humanitarian Crisis in Iraq*. Geneva: ICRC.

———. 2008. *Iraq: No Let Up in the Humanitarian Crisis*. Geneva: ICRC.

International Crisis Group. 2008a. *Failed Responsibility: Iraqi Refugees in Syria, Jordan and Lebanon*. Brussels: International Crisis Group.

———. 2008b. *Oil for Soil: Toward a Grand Bargain on Iraq and the Kurds*. Kirkuk/Brussels: International Crisis Group.

International Organization for Migration (IOM). 2008a. *IDP Working Group: Internally Displaced Persons in Iraq—Update (June 2008)*. New York: IOM.

———. 2008b. *Assessment on Psychosocial Needs of Iraqis Displaced in Jordan and Lebanon*. Amman and Beirut: IOM.

Iraq Body Count. 2009. Retrieved from www.iraqbodycount.org.

———. 2018. Retrieved from www.iraqbodycount.org.

Iraq Family Health Survey Study Group. 2008. "Violence-Related Mortality in Iraq from 2002 to 2006." *New England Journal of Medicine* 358, no. 5: 484–493.

Juhasz, Antonia. 2007. *The Bush Agenda: Invading the World, One Economy at a Time*. New York: Harper Perennial.

Kami, Aseel 2008. "Iraq Tries to Attract Back Doctors Who Fled Violence." *Reuters News Service*. Retrieved from www.reuters.com.

Keen, David J. 2008. *Complex Emergencies*. Malden, MA: Polity Press.

Kim, Jim Yong, Joyce V. Millen, Alec Irwin, and John Gershman, eds. 2002. *Dying for Growth: Global Inequality and the Health of the Poor*. Monroe, ME: Common Courage Press.

Klein, Naomi. 2007. *The Shock Doctrine: The Rise of Disaster Capitalism*. New York: Metropolitan Books.

Krause, Keith, with David Mutimer. 2005. "Introduction." In *Small Arms Survey: Weapons at War*, pp. 1–7. London: Oxford University Press.

Levy, Barry S., and Victor W. Sidel. 2013. "Adverse Health Consequences of the Iraq War." *The Lancet* 381, 949–958.
Libal, Kathryn, and Scott Harding. 2009. "Challenging US Silence: International NGOs and the Iraqi Refugee Crisis." In *International Migration and Human Rights: The Global Repercussions of US Policy*, edited by Samuel Martinez, 216–233. Berkeley: University of California Press.
Lubkemann, Stephen C. 2008. *Culture in Chaos: An Anthropology of the Social Condition of War*. Chicago: University of Chicago Press.
Marfleet, Philip. 2007. "Iraqi Refugees: 'Exit' from the State." *International Journal of Contemporary Iraqi Studies* 1, no. 3: 397–419.
Mattei, Ugo, and Laura Nader. 2008. *Plunder: When the Rule of Law Is Illegal*. Malden, MA: Blackwell.
MedAct. 2004. *Enduring Effects of War: Health in Iraq 2004*. London: MedAct.
———. 2008. *Rehabilitation Under Fire: Health Care in Iraq, 2003–2007*. London: MedAct.
NGO Coordination Committee in Iraq and Oxfam International. 2007. *Rising to the Humanitarian Challenge in Iraq: Briefing Paper 105*. London: Oxfam International.
Nordstrom, C. 2004. *Shadows of War: Violence, Power, and International Profiteering in the Twenty-First Century*. Berkeley: University of California Press.
Opinion Research Business. 2008. "Analysis 'Confirms' 1 Million + Iraq Casualties." Press release. February 15. Retrieved from www.opinion.co.uk.
Oppel, Jr., Richard A. 2006, November 11. "Qaeda Official Is Said to Taunt U.S. on Tape." *New York Times*, A8.
Ostrach, Bayla, and Merrill Singer. 2013. "Syndemics of War: Malnutrition-Infectious Disease Interactions and the Unintended Health Consequences of Intentional Health Policies." *Annals of Anthropological Practice* 36, 2: 257–273. doi:10.1111/napa.12003.
Pedersen, Jon. 2007. "Three Wars Later. Iraqi Living Conditions." In *Iraq: Preventing a New Generation of Conflict*, edited by M. E. Bouillon, D. M. Malone, and B. Rowswell, 55–70. Boulder, CO: Lynne Rienner.
Phillips, David L. 2005. *Losing Iraq: Inside the Postwar Reconstruction Fiasco*. Boulder, CO: Westview Press.
Physicians for Social Responsibility. 2015. *Body Count: Casualty Figures after 10 Years of the "War on Terror."* March. Washington, DC.
Popal, G. R. 2000. "Impact of Sanctions on the Population of Iraq." *Eastern Mediterranean Health Journal* 6, no. 4: 791–795.
Rawaf, Salman. 2005. "The Health Crisis in Iraq." *Critical Public Health* 15, no. 2: 181–188.
Roberts, Les, Riyadh Lafta, Richard Garfield, Jamal Khudhairi, and Gilbert Burnham. 2004. "Mortality Before and After the 2003 Invasion of Iraq: Cluster Sample Survey." *The Lancet* 364, no. 9448: 1857–1864.
Sassoon, Joseph. 2009. *The Iraqi Refugees: The New Crisis in the Middle East*. New York: I.B. Tauris.

———. 2016. "Iraq's Political Economy Post 2003: From Transition to Corruption." *International Journal of Contemporary Iraqi Studies* 10, 1–2: 17–33.

Save the Children. 2007. *State of the World's Mothers 2007. Saving the Lives of Children Under 5.* Westport, CT: Save the Children.

Scheper-Hughes, Nancy, and Philippe Bourgois. 2004. *Violence in War and Peace: An Anthology.* Malden, MA: Wiley-Blackwell Press.

Special Inspector General for Iraq Reconstruction. 2008. *Quarterly Report to the United States Congress, April 30, 2008.* Washington, DC: SIGIR.

Steele, Jonathan, and Susan Goldenberg. 2008. "What Is the Real Death Toll in Iraq?" *Guardian*, March 19.

Susman, Tina. 2007, April 25. "U.N. Report and Times Data Paint Grim Iraq Picture." *Los Angeles Times*.

Susskind, Yifat. 2007. *Promising Democracy, Imposing Theocracy: Gender-Based Violence and the US War on Iraq.* New York: MADRE.

Tirman, John. 2008. "Counting Iraqi Casualties—and a Media Controversy." *Editor and Publisher*, February 14. Retrieved from www.nonviolentworm.org.

United Nations Assistance Mission for Iraq (UNAMI). 2007a. *Human Rights Report 1 November–31 December 2006.* New York: UNAMI.

———. 2007b. *Humanitarian Briefing on the Crisis in Iraq.* New York: UNAMI.

———. 2007c. *Humanitarian Crisis in Iraq: Facts and Figures.* New York: UNAMI.

United Nations Children's Fund (UNICEF). 1998. *Situation Analysis of Children and Women in Iraq.* New York: UNICEF.

———. 2007. *Immediate Needs for Iraqi Children in Iraq and Neighbouring Countries.* Geneva: UNICEF.

———. 2008a. "Sanitation Becoming a Luxury in Iraq." New York: UNICEF. Retrieved from www.unicef.org.

———. 2008b. *Update for Partners on the Situation of Children in Iraq, First Quarter 2008.* Geneva: UNICEF.

United Nations Development Program (UNDP). 2002. *Living Conditions in Iraq.* New York: UNDP.

———. 2008. *Human Development Report: Iraq 2007/2008.* New York: UNDP.

United Nations High Commissioner for Refugees (UNHCR). 2008. *Assessment on Returns to Iraq amongst the Iraqi Refugee Population in Syria.* Geneva: UNHCR.

United Nations World Food Program (UNWFP). 2003. *The Extent and Geographic Distribution of Chronic Poverty in Iraq's Center/South Region.* New York: UNWFP.

———. 2004. *Baseline Food Security Analysis in Iraq.* New York: UNWFP.

United Nations World Food Program (UNWFP)/Central Organization for Statistics and Information Technology (COSIT). 2006. *Food Security and Vulnerability Analysis in Iraq.* Baghdad: UNWFP/COSIT.

Webster, Paul C. 2016. "'Under Severe Duress': Health Care in Iraq." *The Lancet*, 388: 226–227.

World Health Organization (WHO). 2008. "Iraq." Retrieved from www.who.int.

6

The Political Capital of War Wounds

GHASSAN SOLEIMAN ABU-SITTAH

> It is not possible to study the technologies of power without an analysis of the political rationalities ["mentalité"] underpinning them.
> —Thomas Lemke

More than a decade after the American invasion of Iraq, health and medical services in the country remain in tatters. The two American wars and the intervening sanctions have contributed to the death of hundreds of thousands of Iraqis and the affliction of millions over the past twenty years. Crucially as well, Iraq has not been able to recover from the processes that have dismantled the state infrastructure and its capacity to provide care and services to its general population (Rawaf and Rawaf 2012).

With what was the most advanced healthcare system in the Middle East prior to the 1990s, Iraq experienced the exodus of half of its 34,000 medical doctors, the destruction of hospitals, and degradation of medical services (Burnham et al. 2012). Over the past years, tens of thousands of Iraqis have sought their way out of Iraq for medical care, either funded privately or through state-sponsored agreements with regional medical centers. Their itineraries have taken them to Delhi, Beirut, Amman, Tehran, and Istanbul (Dewachi 2013).

The American University of Beirut Medical Center (AUBMC) is the region's oldest regional referral center. Patients from as far as Libya and Yemen come to the AUBMC for specialist treatment. Around 10 percent of the total number of patients come from Iraq. These patients are either privately financed or sent through a bilateral agreement between AUBMC and the Iraqi Ministry of Health.

By their very nature, war injuries are complex, requiring costly, time-consuming, multi-stage, and often expensive surgeries. In terms of both expense and quality, treatment at the AUBMC sits at the pinnacle of medical services available to Iraqi patients. This chapter looks at this population of patients and asks two primary questions: "Why did this particular Iraqi patient (and not any of the hundreds if not thousands like him or worse off) come for treatment at the AUBMC?" and "What was the nature of the selection process by which a chosen few were able to benefit from this expensive and high-profile care?" The answers to these questions will shed light on the various political factors that shape a patient's treatment-seeking behavior, as well as on the factors that determine to what extent that patient will be able to access medical resources.

The biological aim of war is to out-injure and out-kill the enemy. This chapter is based on the premise that, at the moment of infliction, the weapon imparts a narrative onto the body that remains with the war-wounded throughout their lifetime. The narrative of the wound has within it the story of that war (why, where, and by whom, if the perpetrators are known). This narrative, which may not change in the official telling, is known intrinsically by the wounded, who, in the telling of their stories, often emphasize it or downplay it if it has become useless in the present day. However, from the moment of infliction, the war wound carries a certain political capital: Power elites determine the value of this capital based on the degree to which the political narrative of the wound concords with or contradicts their current political project. The political value of the wound will vary during the lifetime of the injured with the changing fortunes of political projects and the elite that carried those projects. This political value becomes the main determinant of access to healthcare.

Methodology

This chapter builds upon the author's experience as a plastic and reconstructive surgeon for seven years at AUBMC and as the co-director of the Conflict Medicine Program. Case studies from the author's own experience during these years will be examined against existing literature on the historical processes of the Iraq wars.

Case Studies: The History of Iraq through Its War Wounds

Seldom has there been a country like Iraq, which has seen so much political upheaval, each chapter of which has left a pathological imprint of literally millions of war wounds in the lifetime of a single generation. A history of these wars must be told in order to better understand these war wounds and their respective prognoses.

The Iraq-Iran War

The armed conflict between the Islamic Republic of Iran and the Republic of Iraq lasted from September 1980 to August 1988, making it the twentieth century's longest conventional war. Estimates of war deaths vary. The Battle Deaths Dataset estimates direct combat fatalities at more than 600,000 in Iraq. The Correlates of War Project, another major scholarly dataset, put the number at 500,000 Iraqi and 750,000 Iranian dead (Kurzman 2013).

It is difficult to estimate the number of Iraqis injured in this war. Mohammad Esfandiari, director of communications and public relations of Iran's Martyrs and Disabled Veterans' Organization, announced the latest numbers of surviving veterans as of June 2014: 548,499 disabled veterans of the Iraq-Iran war are currently living in Iran (Samimi 2014). Yet what is known is that, until the fall of Saddam Hussain's regime and the US occupation in 2003, Iraq's injured were considered to be heroes of what was termed "Saddam's *Qaddisiyah*," Saddam's invocation of Arab nationalism in opposition to the Persian sentiment at the time. As such, they had access to the best that Iraq's health sector could offer. The Ministry of Defense gave veterans with permanent disabilities specially built accessible housing, and a factory owned by the Ministry of Defense provided them with prosthetic limbs.

This all ended in 2003. The Iraqi Army was disbanded by the US-appointed Interim Government. Political parties that had sided with Iran during the war came to power, and the new Iraqi government formally apologized to the Islamic Republic of Iran for starting what it called "Saddam's war of aggression." In a related move, the Iraqi government removed the honorific descriptor "martyr" from Iraqi soldiers killed in the Iraq-Iran war. This resulted in the loss of benefits to previously named "martyrs," including the loss of pension, the loss of both financial subsidies and preferential access to the social welfare state, and the loss of those benefits for their children. In addition, the new government no longer gave the injured from the Iran-Iraq war priority in medical treatment or referred them to regional hospitals for expensive tertiary treatment. The old narrative about their war wounds—that they were suffered at the hands of Iran, the mortal enemy not only Iraq and Iraqis, but of the Arab nation as a whole—stood in stark contrast with the political narrative of the new Iraqi regime, which saw in Iran a political and ideological ally. Meanwhile, the new Iraqi parliament voted on legislation known as the Jihad Service Law, offering wide privileges, including advanced medical care, to the members of the newly dominant political parties for the years they spent fighting the former regime, some of them alongside Iranian troops (Mamouri 2014).

The 2003 American Invasion and Occupation of Iraq

At a minimum, according to Brown University's Costs of War Project, 165,000 civilians were recorded killed by war's violence between 2003 and 2013 in Iraq. But many deaths in Iraq were unreported or unrecorded: Thus, this number, based on tallies of government and press reports, is an undercount (Crawford 2015). According to Iraq Body Count (IBC), the one organization that attempted to document all of the war's violent deaths in Iraq, full recording of Iraqi violent deaths would show a toll of 251,000 civilians and combatants, also estimating a higher number of deaths than those reported (Iraq Body Count 2016). Thus, the toll of violent death due to war may exceed 250,000 people.

The number of seriously injured Iraqi men, women, and children in the war was about the same as those killed. The Iraq war produced the kinds of casualties associated with every war—direct deaths and injuries due to combat-related violence; violent deaths and injuries due to lawlessness following the breakdown of the state, e.g., revenge killing; deaths due to accidents related to military occupation, such as traffic crashes caused by military convoys or at checkpoints; and the indirect deaths that result from the destruction of infrastructure and the lingering environmental effects of war (Crawford 2015).[1]

Civilians are wounded in the same way that they are killed: in cross fire; in bombings; by improvised explosive devices; and by suicide bombs. Injury rates vary by weapon and method: For instance, the injured to killed ratio for civilians by suicide bomb was 2.5 injured to every one person killed (Hicks et al. 2011). Similarly, the US National Counterterrorism Center, which focuses only on "terrorist" events, counted about 110,000 wounded Iraqis from 2004 through 2010 (US National Counterterrorism Center 2011). The Iraq Body Count dataset does include wounds caused by all parties, but it only tallied incidents where at least one civilian death occurred; incidents where there are only injuries, but no deaths, were not recorded.

According to a 2010 report by Handicap International, 13,000 cluster munitions, containing 1.8 to 2 million sub-munitions, were used by the United States and Britain in 2003 in the first weeks of combat, and as a result Iraq remains one of the most heavily contaminated countries with unexploded ammunition, including mines, in the world (Cluster Munition Coalition 2010, 3). Centers supported by the International Committee for the Red Cross provided more than 300 prostheses for survivors of mines to Iraqis in 2009. The ICRC noted that, "The series of conflicts that took place in Iraq and the ongoing turmoil there, together with the still weak public health-care system, resulted in an ever-growing number of disabled people. Unfortunately, there was still no way to pinpoint that number with certainty." But the ICRC noted that the need for orthotic support devices and prostheses would grow, even assuming no more are wounded (ICRC 2009, 62). "The WHO's estimate that 0.5 percent of the total population was in need of physical rehabilitation would put the figure at 156,000; since all of them would need a new orthopedic device every three years on average, this would mean an average annual production of over 52,000 devices" (ibid.).

The Iraqi Civil War

Following the 2003 US-launched invasion of Iraq, intercommunal violence between Iraqi Sunni and Shi'a factions became prevalent. In February 2006, al Qaeda in Iraq bombed one of the holiest sites in Shi'a Islam—the al-Askari Mosque in Samarra. This set off a wave of Shi'a reprisals against Sunnis, followed by Sunni counterattacks. The conflict escalated over the next several months until, by 2007, the National Intelligence Estimate described the situation as having elements of a civil war. In 2008 and 2009, the violence declined dramatically. On the Shi'a side, militias linked to political parties in the Iraqi government carried out reprisals. However, the Iraqi regime's narrative held that the violence was being perpetrated against all Iraqis regardless of sect and that al Qaeda in Iraq was perpetrating all the violence.

In 2009, the Iraqi government ratified a law entitled "Compensating the Victims of Military Operations, Military Mistakes and Terrorist Actions (the Compensation Law)," which regulated the payment of compensation for those who suffered from acts of violence. It formed a governmental committee to accept applications from beneficiaries, and subsequently opened branches in most provinces. These branches predominated in the southern governorates where the majority of Saddam's victims are located and where the power bases of the new political elites lay.

Critically, the law excludes those killed by American forces during the invasion and occupation and the victims of militias whose political parties are represented on the compensation committee, in addition to those injured in the Iraq-Iran war. It considers as victims of terrorism only those injured by acts perpetrated by al Qaeda.

Iraqi Ministry of Interior versus the Ministry of Defense

The American occupation forces disbanded the Iraqi Army. The army they set up in its place was less well equipped and trained, and it transferred the job of internal security to the Ministry of Interior with its Federal Police Force. The Ministry of Interior eventually grew to be one of the main power bases of the Maliki government, with the Federal Police Force growing to 750,000 strong with the help of extensive US reconstruction funding. While Iraqi soldiers injured by terrorist attacks were entitled to compensation only through the Victims of Terrorism act, those requiring treatment abroad had to apply through the Ministry of Health's mechanism for treating all Iraqis abroad. In addition, the Ministry of Interior had a multimillion "Martyrs Fund." It signed bilateral agreements with regional health centers in Jordan, Lebanon, India,

Iran, and Turkey supervised by its own medical corps (Dewachi 2015). It set about building hospitals to be run by its medical corps, while it never reconstituted the Iraqi Army's medical corps.

The Rise of ISIS and the Defeat of the Iraqi Police by the Iraqi Army

This building process all came to a complete halt when ISIS took over large swaths of northern Iraq, leading to the collapse of the Maliki government. A stronger Iraqi Army became a national and international political necessity and with it the need to weaken Maliki's power base at the Ministry of Interior. The new Abadi government abolished the Martyrs Fund, which the Commission of Integrity then referred to the courts. In its place, the new government passed a law establishing the "Martyrs Foundation" with the express aim of supporting not only the army but also the clans and militia fighting ISIS, with no mention of medical support for the Ministry of Interior's Federal Police.

Mapping Iraq's War Injuries across Its Recent Political History

In my professional experience, I have encountered many cases that highlight the tension between the political value of war injuries assigned by power elites at a given time, on one hand, and patients' ability to access medical care, on the other. They illustrate how the political value of injuries has fluctuated over time and during the different conflicts that have taken place over Iraq's recent history. These cases will be discussed with reference to Iraq's changing historical circumstances.

In 2012, an Iraqi male in his late fifties who had been diagnosed with gallstones by ultrasound was referred by the general surgeons at AUBMC for review. The patient was referred because he had lost the majority of his abdominal wall musculature as a direct result of a blast injury. A skin graft had been laid on top of the abdominal cavity. Any attempt at surgically removing his gallbladder would leave him with an open abdominal cavity. The general surgeons were of the opinion that we (Abu-Sittah and surgeons) should take advantage of the fact that the stones were not for the moment causing obstruction and inflammation of the gallbladder, and so we should reconstruct his abdominal wall to make it possible for any future elective or emergency cholecystectomy (removal of the gallbladder) to be safely performed. Upon further history-taking, which required a bit of prompting, it became apparent that the initial injury to the abdominal wall was the result of a blast injury sustained in the first few months of the Iraq-Iran war and that the patient had been operated on by the foreign medical teams the then-government of Iraq had brought in to operate on injured soldiers. The problem was that he was not currently entitled to any state-funded treatment as his injury had taken place during the Iraq-Iran war and current policy is for state subvention only of "terrorism"-related injuries. He had funded his trip to the AUBMC himself but did not have sufficient funds for the reconstruction. He returned home without it.

In another case, a male patient in his mid-thirties presented in 2011 with a large bony defect in the lower jaw. The defect was the aftermath of having been shot by American forces during the occupation as he drove his truck between Iraq and Jordan. The patient was immediately suspected of being an Iraqi insurgent because he was Sunni and he had been shot by American forces, and this had caused him to lose his livelihood as a general trader. He had received care in Syria for three months, as the Ministry of Health had rejected his requests for treatment at AUBMC. One year after the injury, he managed to fund the trip to Beirut himself. He needed reconstruction of his jaw but did not have sufficient funds to pay for the surgery. His clan chief, who was himself a victim of an American bombing raid, eventually paid for the surgery.

These two cases highlight the tension between the narrative of each wound and the dominant political value given to the wound at the time of treatment. Pre-2003, the wounded of the Iraq-Iran war had been celebrated as national heroes, and all resources available to the Iraqi state had been devoted to the care and treatment of these injured. Following the 2003 American invasion, the Iraq-Iran war was viewed as one of Saddam's crimes against both the Iraqi and Iranian people, and the wounded, once lauded as heroes, became an embarrassment to the Iraq that was now allied with Iran. At the same time, after the American invasion, Iraqis injured by American forces have faced a similar problem, in that their wounds and their need for ongoing care contradict the narrative of the elite currently ruling Iraq. In both cases, the political capital of the wounds carried a "negative" value, which translated into these patients' inability to access healthcare.

During the Iraqi Civil War, on the other hand, the war-injured whose narrative was in line with that of the religious authorities who made up the political elite of the time were more likely to access treatment for their wounds than soldiers or civilians who had been caught up in the civil strife. For example, a patient who was operating heavy machinery on a construction project to expand the holy sites in Karbala, Iraq, was injured in the leg by a secondary explosive device aimed at individuals coming to aid those injured by a primary bomb in Karbala in 2007. He was immediately airlifted to Beirut and the religious authorities who ran the holy sites paid for the entirety of his medical treatment, which involved complex microsurgical reconstruction and cost approximately $60,000.

A businessman in his early thirties presented acutely with a forefoot amputation secondary to a magnetic bomb (a bomb attached by a magnet to the car undercarriage) placed underneath his car during the civil strife. Unlike the heavy machinery operator, his first trip and subsequent surgeries were all self-funded. His business was in an area of Baghdad that was the target of communal cleansing by the Shi'a militias whose political parties currently run the Ministry of Health.

Cases of discrepancies between different war-injured patients and their ability to access treatment also varied before the takeover of Mosul by ISIS and after. Cases before the takeover of Mosul were covered by the Ministry of Interior's Martyrs Fund, which was the power base of the Maliki government. For example, in 2012 a police officer in his late thirties who was manning a checkpoint in front of the Ministry of Interior noticed a man acting suspiciously. As the officer approached him, the man ran toward the crowds; but before he was able to detonate his vest, the officer threw himself on the man and his bomb went off. The officer sustained a severely mangled left leg. The Undersecretary of the Ministry of Interior refused to allow the doctors to amputate and ordered his transfer to Beirut. By the time he returned to Iraq three months later, having completed his limb salvage and reconstruction surgeries, his medical bill, all paid for by the Ministry of Interior's Martyrs Fund, stood at $200,000. Around the same time, and well before the takeover of Mosul, a soldier who had been manning a checkpoint in Diwaniyah in central Iraq when a suicide bomber detonated presented at the AUBMC. His injury had left him with severe facial deformity and the loss of both eyes. He received compensation upon discharge from the army of just $700 and had to pay out of pocket for his facial reconstructive surgery, which cost $15,000; he had to wait until two years after the injury in order to save adequate personal funds.

Since the takeover of Mosul, all patients referred by the Ministry of Health to the AUBMC's reconstructive surgery services have been members of the Iraqi Army. Previously, the Ministry of Health by and large sent civilians. In the first six months following the takeover, the AUBMC had treated more than one hundred officers and soldiers, with gunshots and blast injuries, all paid for by the Iraqi Ministry of Health.

A nineteen-year-old member of *Al-Hashd*, the militia formed by religious decree from Ayatollah al-Sistani to fight ISIS alongside the Iraqi Army, was shot in the leg by an ISIS sniper on the outskirts of Fallujah. Within days of his injury, he was transferred to Beirut to undergo the first stage of his limb salvage surgery. The newly formed Martyrs Foundation, established by the Abadi government, paid for both the initial and subsequent trips. The Al-Hashd militia was critical to the Iraqi government and religious authorities' attempts to rally the population to their call to fight ISIS and was viewed as exemplifying the popular response to the religious authority's call to arms.

These cases illustrate how, even within the same political elite, the rise and fall of different wings within this elite (such as the fall of the Maliki government and the demise of its stronghold, and the emergence of Al-Hashd and the Iraqi Army as the two forces fighting ISIS) translates into different political value ascribed to the wounds. Each change in political project brings with it a change in the value of the political capital of each wound. As illustrated by the above case studies, that change in political value can have a dramatic and sometimes severe impact on the war wound itself and its prognosis.

Conclusion

At the moment of infliction, the weapon imparts a narrative onto the body that remains with the war-wounded for his lifetime. The narrative of the wound is the political narrative of the war and has within it the story of that war (why, where, and by whom). This narrative cannot be changed and thus has to be either emphasized or subjugated depending on the value ascribed to it by the current power elite. Power elites determine the political value based on the degree to which the narrative of the wound concords with or contradicts their current political project. The political value of the war wound will vary during the lifetime of the injured with the changing fortunes of political projects and the elite that carried them and is the main determinant of access to healthcare.

In his essay, "Ideology and Ideological State Apparatuses (Notes Towards an Investigation)," French Marxist philosopher Louis Althusser theorized the process of identification through which individuals become "knowing subjects" (Althusser 1971). Althusser theorized the process of hailing, that is, the process of the constitution of the individual as subject within language and ideology, as fundamental to human societies. In Althusser's theorization, the process of recognition by the individual of herself or himself as the one addressed by the call to recognition *interpellates* the individual as a subject within ideology. This process of identification, Althusser argued, inserts individuals into ideologies and ideological practices that, when they work well, are lived as if they were obvious and natural. According to Althusser, a range of what he terms "Ideological State Apparatuses," such as religion, education, family, law, politics, culture, and media, produces the ideologies within which we assume identities and become subjects. The value ascribed to the war wound by political elites reaches its pinnacle when the narrative of the wound is in complete concordance with the current political project of the power elite. At this point the war wound becomes a form of *biointerpellation*, its narrative placing it within the dominant ideology.

At the opposite end of the value spectrum (negative equity), the narrative of the war wound will completely contradict, if not potentially delegitimize, the political project of the dominant elites. This requires subjugation of the war wound and its narrative. The exclusion of knowledge from below is what Michel Foucault in his book *Discipline and Punish: The Birth of a Prison* (1979) calls *subjugated knowledge*. Briefly defined, it is: "local, discontinuous, disqualified, illegitimate knowledges." Power is realized and knowledge is placed in a subordinate position through discourses. There is a tug-of-war between discourses; they interact with each other, but also influence who can speak, what can be said, and when it can be said. Certain discourses dominate over others because they favor versions of social reality that justify existing social structures and power relations. When the narrative of the wound contradicts the dominant version of social and political reality, its narrative is subjugated, and one of the mechanisms of subjugation is ascribing a negative political value to it, where the wound is often ignored, untreated, and not paid for.

The phenomenon described is not limited to Iraq or the AUBMC. The continuous upheaval in Iraq over the past thirty years and the position of the AUBMC within the region's health systems have allowed us to see more clearly the process by which different dominant elites, at different times, give value to the political capital imbued within war wounds because this value is expressed in tangible monetary terms.

While the health consequences of war injuries often remain for the lifetime of patients and their need for medical care increases with the aging process, the political value given to their wound is always temporal. The majority of the injured will outlive the dominant elites and political projects that gave a high political value to their wounds. The wounds of the patient injured in the Iraq-Iran war have outlived Saddam and his regime, the Soviet Union, Ayatollah Khomeini, and President Reagan. Prior to the fall of Saddam Hussein, one patient's wound was sufficiently politically valuable that a foreign medical team was brought to Iraq to operate on him and others like him. Yet in his lifetime, he has seen the political capital of his wound devalue, as it ended up on the wrong side of the current dominant elite's political agenda. The temporal nature of this political capital is not only because it is the product of the identity of dominant elites but also their political projects. The changing fortunes of members of Iraq's Ministry of Interior vis-à-vis those from the Iraqi Army, before and after the takeover of Mosul, show how changing political priorities within the same elite are reflected in the value they give to the wound.

Discrepancies in healthcare access among the various Iraqi war wounded transcend other forms of discrimination in access to healthcare such as those based on class, ethnic, or religious identities and is the main determinant of access to healthcare needed to treat war wounds. The decision as to whether to cheaply amputate an injured lower limb at a local hospital or to send the patient abroad for lengthy and expensive reconstruction depends not on the traditional forms of identity markers of the injured such as socioeconomic status or sectarian identity, but instead depends on the narrative of the war wound and the political value this generates. None of the "Injury Severity Scores"[2] designed to help surgeons predict which lower limb injury is salvageable include an anthropological narrative of the wound as one the determinants of outcome, yet as we have tried to demonstrate, they should. Access to reconstructive technology and expertise comes at great expense. This cost is only met when the political value of the wound is worth the price.

Neither is this phenomenon limited to the tragedy of Iraq. The injured of the Great Patriotic War have gone from being heroes of the USSR, to the neglected remnants of the Soviet past during the Yeltsin years, and back again at the heart of Putin's imperial project. American sub-stratification of war wounds grades them according to their assigned political value and not severity of injury. For example, while those hit directly by ordnance are considered Grade 1 injuries, those hit by collision with the second vehicle during an ambush are classified as Grade III (Defense Finance and Accounting Services 2015). Dominant elites treat war wounds as the biological embodiment of political projects. They will always seek the legitimation inherent in the narrative of some war wounds or try to bury them.

NOTES

1 Three studies have examined the effects of the war and sanctions on Iraqi civilians. The first *Lancet* study, published in 2004, estimated that about 98,000 excess deaths (over what could be expected if Iraq had not been at war) had occurred in Iraq from March 19, 2003 to September 16, 2004. The second *Lancet* study, published in 2006, gave a range of between 426,000 and 793,000 killed after the invasion through July 2006 (Sloboda, Dougherty, and Dardagan 2007, 7). More specifically, the authors estimated about 655,000 excess deaths, of which they suggested some 601,000 were due to violent causes. A study published in the *New England Journal of Medicine*, conducted by the Iraq Family Health Survey Study Group, surveyed a larger number of household clusters than *The Lancet* published studies, but found a lower number of violent deaths; they estimated 151,000 deaths from March 2003 to June 2006 (Burnham et al. 2006). An even higher figure for violent death—more than one million killed—was given in 2007 by the Opinion Research Bureau (ORB), based in Britain (Iraq Family Health Survey Study Group et al. 2008).

2 Injury Severity Scores (ISS) are used in reconstructive surgery and are designed to help determine whether a limb needs amputation. These scores are based on physiological data, such as amount of blood lost, nerve damage, etc.

REFERENCES

Althusser, Louis. 1971. "Ideology and Ideological State Apparatuses (Notes towards an Investigation)." In *Lenin and Philosophy and Other Essays*, edited by Louis Althusser. New York: Monthly Review Press.

Burnham, Gilbert, Riyadh Lafta, Shannon Doocy, and Les Roberts. 2006. "Mortality after the 2003 Invasion of Iraq: A Cross-sectional Cluster Sample Survey." *The Lancet* 368 (9545): 1421–28.

Burnham, Gilbert, Sana Malik, Ammar S. Al-Shibli, Ali Rasheed Mahjoub, Alya'a Qays Baqer, Zainab Qays Baqer, Faraj Al Qaraghuli, and Shannon Doocy. 2012. "Understanding the Impact of Conflict on Health Services in Iraq: Information from 401 Iraqi Refugee Doctors in Jordan." *International Journal of Health Planning and Management* 27 (1): e51–64.

Cluster Munition Coalition. 2010. *Cluster Munition Monitor 2010*. Canada: Mines Action Canada.

Crawford, Neta. 2015. "Civilian Death and Injury in the Iraq War, 2003–2013." Retrieved from http://watson.brown.edu/costsofwar.

Defense Finance and Accounting Services. 2015. "Combat Related Special Compensation." Retrieved from www.dfas.mil.

Dewachi, Omar. 2013. "War and the Costs of Medical Travel for Iraqis in Lebanon." Retrieved from http://watson.brown.edu/costsofwar.

———. 2015. "When Wounds Travel." *Medicine Anthropology Theory* 2 (3): 61–82.

Foucault, Michel. 1979. *Discipline and Punish: The Birth of a Prison*. New York: Vintage Books.

Hicks, Madelyn Hsiao-Rei, Hamit Dardagan, Peter M. Bagnall, Michael Spagat, and John A. Sloboda. 2011. "Casualties in Civilians and Coalition Soldiers from Suicide Bombings in Iraq, 2003–10: A Descriptive Study." *The Lancet* 378 (9794): 906–14.

International Committee for the Red Cross. 2009. *Physical Rehabilitation Programme, Annual Report 2009*. Geneva: ICRC.

Iraq Body Count. 2016. "Iraq Body Count." Retrieved from www.iraqbodycount.org.

Iraq Family Health Survey Study Group, Amir H. Alkhuzai, Ihsan J. Ahmad, Mohammed J. Hweel, Thakir W. Ismail, Hanan H. Hasan, Abdul Rahman Younis, Osman Shawani, Vian M. Al-Jaf, Mahdi M. Al-Alak, Louay H. Rasheed, Suham M. Hamid, Naeema Al-Gasseer, Fazia A. Majeed, Naira A. Al Awqati, Mohamed M. Ali, J. Ties Boerma, and Colin Mathers. 2008. "Violence-related Mortality in Iraq from 2002 to 2006." *New England Journal of Medicine* 358 (5): 484–93.

Kurzman, Charles. 2013. "Death Tolls of the Iran-Iraq War." *UNC: Charles Kurzman*, October 31.

Mamouri, Ali. 2014. "Transitional Justice Fails in Iraq." *Al-Monitor*, June 6.

Rawaf, Salman, and David Rawaf. 2012. "Public Health in Crisis: Iraq." In *Public Health in the Arab World*, edited by Samer Jabbour, Rita Giacaman, Marwan Khawaja, and Iman Nuwayhid. Cambridge: Cambridge University Press.

Samimi, Mehrnaz. 2014. "Iran's Disabled Veterans Lack Services, Access." *Al-Monitor*, September 29.

Sloboda, John, Josh Dougherty, and Hamit Dardagan. 2007. "The State of Knowledge on Civilian Casualties in Iraq: Counts, Estimates, and Government Responsibility." *Iraq Body Count*. Retrieved from www.iraqbodycount.org.

US National Counterterrorism Center (NCTC). 2011. "Worldwide Incidents Tracking System." Retrieved from wits.nctc.gov.

7

Iraqis' Cancer Itineraries

War, Medical Travel, and Therapeutic Geographies

MAC SKELTON

Coinciding with dips in Beirut's tourism industry over the past decade, a cluster of hotels in the vicinity of the city's hospitals have increasingly relied upon a new source of business: Iraqis traveling to Lebanon for medical treatments of various kinds, particularly cancer care. At a one-star establishment located a few hundred meters from Beirut's main oncology center, Iraqis seeking cancer care have consistently occupied a majority of the rooms since 2007. Wheelchairs are stacked at the entrance, and TVs are often tuned to Iraqi news channels. Hotel employees assist patients with their IVs, while patients and relatives recline on the couches near the main entrance after long days of treatments.

Much of the conversation revolves around difficulties in securing funds for chemotherapy, tests, and MRIs. Due to the long temporality and cyclical management of cancer, it is common for patients to go back and forth between Iraq and Lebanon, returning to the hotel with each new trip for care. Located a few city blocks away, a three-star hotel has focused on a niche business: medical delegations funded by the Iraqi Ministry of Health (IMOH). Patients and family-member escorts occupy nearly every room on multiple floors of this hotel, where they reside free of charge, with all bills paid by IMOH. At mealtimes, they descend to the subcontracted restaurant next door, submit a white slip of paper, and receive a dish of their choice. The Lebanese hospital contracted by the IMOH communicates with the hotel reception desk regarding appointments.

While Iraq once boasted the Middle East's strongest medical system, decades of wars and sanctions have led to a mass exodus of doctors and the deterioration of health facilities. In addition to Iraqi refugees and displaced persons who rely heavily on the healthcare systems of neighboring countries, families living in Iraq have, since 2003, increasingly pooled resources and traveled temporarily for treatments in Lebanon, Turkey, Iran, Jordan, and even India. Iraqis board planes and travel internationally for cataract removal, cardiac surgeries, and chemotherapy, among other treatments. Self-funded treatment itineraries overlap with government-sponsored delegations. The IMOH has contracted with hospitals in regional countries to administer treatments that the Baghdad-based ministry can no longer provide, including complex procedures such as bone marrow transplants for leukemia (Iraqi Ministry of Health 2014) and reconstructive surgeries for blast injuries (Anderson 2015). In cafes and hotels throughout Beirut's medical district, both self-funded patients and government-sponsored care-seekers intermingle and exchange advice about doctors, medical reports, and even mortuary services. Similar forms of sociality can be observed among Iraqis traveling for treatments in Istanbul and New Delhi. What can scholars make of these transnational movements for care under conditions of war?

Based on fieldwork in Lebanon and the Kurdish region of Iraq,[1] this chapter focuses specifically on how Iraqis traveling for cancer care navigate this emerging geography. Whereas Baghdad was the unquestioned national hub for chemotherapy and radiotherapy prior to 1991, a growing cancer burden among the Iraqi population, combined with the exodus of medical specialists over the course of multiple US-led military campaigns, has reduced the centrality of the capital city and led to the emergence of new national and regional hubs for Iraqi patients seeking cancer care.[2] These include domestic sites such as Erbil and Sulaimani, located in the relatively stable Kurdish region of Iraq, as well as regional centers for oncology such as those in Beirut, Amman, and Istanbul.

Academic interest in patients moving for care internationally gained momentum in the late 1980s and 1990s as scholarly attention to "medical tourism" grew and focused on the rapid growth of health tourism in countries endowed with thermal springs and other natural resources viewed as healing agents (Niv 1989; Even-Paz and Shani 1989; Kevan 1993). Soon, however, broader concerns emerged. "Medical tourism" became a term that encompassed not only natural therapies but also biomedical ones, and thus scholars debated the impact of growing medical tourism on national healthcare systems (Carrera and Bridges

2006). Coinciding with increased discussion of globalization in the social sciences (Appadurai 1996), researchers analyzed medical tourism as a product of the globalization of medicine and the emergence of "patients without borders" (Ramírez de Arellano 2007). When anthropologists studying the Middle East started to engage these conversations, they challenged the language of the existing literature, namely, the usage of the term "medical tourism" (Inhorn 2011; Kangas 2010). They problematized that term on the grounds that poor or limited local health infrastructure often leaves patients with no alternative other than international travel for life-saving treatment, including oncology. For instance, Kangas (2010) highlights how deficiencies in local oncology services give Yemeni patients no other choice but to travel abroad to Jordan and elsewhere. One of Kangas's primary concerns is the question of financial resources. She rejects the notion that "only wealthy and well-connected seek treatment abroad" (2010, 348). While some families are able to access corporate support for treatment in Jordan, many rely exclusively on kinship networks and sell belongings to fund treatment and travel (ibid.). Thus, "medical travel" or "therapeutic journeys" are preferable terms as they remove the assumed association between medical tourism and "leisure" (Kangas 2010, 350–354). This shift in terminology has aimed to maintain the centrality of movement for care without perpetuating faulty assumptions around the circumstances, contexts, or experiences of that movement.[3]

How does medical travel appear in a context where war has reshaped the national and regional dynamics of healthcare? What specific strategies and financial resources enable families to attempt care-seeking trajectories across international borders under conditions of war? Dewachi et al.'s (2014) concept of a "therapeutic geography"—i.e., the geographical redistribution of healthcare under conditions of war—provides a helpful framework for answering these questions within the appropriate historical and political context. Dewachi et al. (2014) argue that wars in Syria and Iraq have generated massive displacements of both populations and medical personnel across borders, and the geography of healthcare in the region has shifted accordingly (ibid., 452). Instead of limiting the impacts of war on healthcare systems to the destruction of infrastructures, therapeutic geographies call for historical and ethnographic exploration of how recent wars in the region have transformed and shaped the movements of patients and trajectories of care-seekers. From this perspective, the rising phenomenon of cancer-related travel between Iraq and neighboring countries indexes broader war-induced transformations in the geographic distribution of healthcare.

The argument proceeds in two parts. After providing a brief overview of the war-related conditions that have generated these shifts in the regional geography of oncology over the past twenty-five years, I turn to two case studies of Iraqis traveling for cancer care. In engaging these cases, the analysis builds on recent research that stresses the importance of exploring how lived experience informs our understanding of therapeutic geographies (Parkinson and Behrouzan 2015). Tracking shifting treatment destinations and accumulating medical fees exposes the contingencies and struggles of medical travel across an emerging therapeutic geography.

Historical Context

Cancer and oncology have been central to the history and politics of recent wars in Iraq. During the 1991 aerial campaign over Iraq, the United States utilized approximately 340 tons of missiles containing depleted uranium (DU) (Peterson 2000). In the years that followed, a DU controversy emerged. Iraqi Health Under Secretary Shawqi Sabri Murcos stated at a 1998 conference in Baghdad: "The use of depleted uranium has caused irreparable damage to Iraq's people and its environment . . . Our surveys show a dramatic increase in cases of leukemia, especially among children in areas of southern Iraq bombed by the allies" (Ciment 1998).[4] The post-1990 destruction of the state oncology infrastructure heightened the stakes of the controversy over DU. It is widely documented that Iraq boasted the Middle East's strongest healthcare system prior to the Gulf War of 1990–1991, and Mula-Hussain (2012) has detailed the long-standing technical excellence and strong expertise of oncology services in particular. While UN sanctions technically exempted medicine and food from the comprehensive import ban, in reality both suffered dramatically. In 1996, an international team of researchers reported that Iraq had one-third fewer hospital beds than when the sanctions began; that hospital stays had been cut in half; and that more than 50 percent of diagnostic and therapeutic equipment in hospitals was no longer functioning due to an absence of spare parts or of maintenance (Garfield, Zaidi, and Lennock 1997).

Sanctions placed especially stringent restrictions on oncology-related imports. The WHO Cancer Program director visited Baghdad in 1999 and noted: "Requested radiotherapy equipment, chemotherapy drugs, and analgesics are consistently blocked by United States and British advisers. There seems to be a rather ludicrous notion that such agents could be converted into chemical or other weapons." Sikora noted "staggering deficiencies in cancer treatment facilities because of the United Nations sanctions" (Sikora 1999). During the 1990s and early 2000s, cancer patients were forced to rely on black markets to supplement hospital provisions of key medications. In the aftermath of the 2003 invasion, supplies for cancer medications dwindled further due to the tightening of border controls and the disruption of distribution channels. Humanitarian aid organizations and American military hospitals frequently turned cancer patients away due to the prioritization of conflict injuries (Duffy 2003).

Since 2003, initiatives to improve oncology services have struggled to gain traction within a broader context in which urban centers were, following the logics of the US-led war on terror, transformed into theaters of war. During the Occupation, Allied forces blurred the lines between combatant and non-combatant, frequently raiding private homes in search of what they identified as insurgents. In this new geography of violence, hospitals, formerly safe havens, often became targets and instruments of war by various parties to the conflict. Doctors and patients were targeted for killings and kidnappings, and trust in the medical system eroded (Dewachi et al. 2014). One report stated that 8,000 of 17,000 doctors had fled from 2003 to 2008 largely due to the danger of assassination (MedAct 2008).

The exodus of doctors as well as persistent gaps in equipment and medications have exacerbated wait times for oncology treatment, which is exclusively provided by state-run hospitals.[5] State doctors commonly encourage patients to travel abroad where they can receive private care and avoid the long queues in Iraqi hospitals, which often involve waits of several months. The scale at which Iraqis are turning down free-of-cost oncology provided by the Iraqi state and traveling elsewhere is striking. According to the lead oncologist of one of Beirut's top cancer centers, 20 percent of all new admissions and 60 percent of daily visits now involve Iraqis traveling to the city for treatment—up from a negligible number just twelve years ago. The medical attaché at the Iraqi Embassy in Beirut claims that tracking the total number of cancer patients arriving to Beirut is impossible as they are spread across dozens of hospitals and rarely register with the Embassy.[6] The only citywide marker currently available is from Beirut's largest mortuary service: It now processes upwards of 250 Iraqi cancer deaths annually for transport back to Iraq. The owner told me during an interview in 2015: "I used to have like one, two or five [Iraqis] a year. Now it's nearly every day. They're all the same, cancer of the stomach, cancer of the lungs, cancer." During my initial period of fieldwork in 2012, the first patient I tracked made several trips back and forth between Beirut and Baghdad before passing away of liver cancer in a Beirut hospital. The family paid $1,500 to the mortuary service in addition to the expensive hospital bills for end-of-life care.

Lebanon's American University of Beirut Medical Center (AUBMC) and Jordan's King Hussein Cancer Center top the list in terms of regional popularity among Iraqi care-seekers. Beyond the Arab states, private hospitals in Tehran, Istanbul, and even New Delhi have also become important destinations. For Iraqi care-seekers desiring an alternative option within the national healthcare system, the public hospitals under the jurisdiction of the semi-autonomous Kurdish Regional Government (KRG) have increasingly received Arab patients traveling from Baghdad, Salah-a-din, and even the southern provinces of Basra and Najaf. As the KRG Ministry of Health receives funds and medications from the Baghdad-based IMOH, its hospital system is legally bound to serve Iraqi citizens regardless of whether they are Kurdish or Arab. Nanakali Cancer Hospital in Erbil and Hiwa Cancer Hospital in Sulaimani have both reported dramatic increases in non-Kurdish patients, including both displaced persons and medical travelers. Wait times have extended significantly as a result of this influx and the limitations of supplies. The current economic downturn due to the sharp decline in the international price paid for Iraqi oil has led to further reductions in medications and funds from the IMOH. It is not uncommon for KRG oncologists to explain the full range of therapeutic options available in different neighboring countries as part of the consultation interview given the lengthy wait times locally.[7]

The Iraqi Ministry of Health has facilitated cross-border movements for select groups of patients through contracts with private hospitals in Lebanon, Turkey, Jordan, and India. These arrangements have proven highly unstable and have been subject to accusations of corruption (Al-Ta'I 2015). In the case study analysis below, we will follow the story of a patient who underwent a government-sponsored bone marrow transplant in Lebanon during the summer of 2014. The patient's timing was fortunate: The bone marrow transplant contract was terminated prematurely later that year. The Iraqi Ministry of Health reduced funding for medical delegations as part of the aforementioned austerity measures.

Not all categories of patients have been impacted equally, however. The increasing prioritization of national security has been reflected in the composition of medical delegations.

In an April 2015 meeting between the Minister of Health and former Prime Minister Nouri Al Maliki, a key point of discussion was the importance of accelerating the medical evacuation of the "heroes" (*abtal*) injured in the campaign against ISIS, including the "armed forces" as well as those from the *Hashd Shaabi* (Popular Mobilization Forces).[8] Medical delegations arriving to Beirut are increasingly comprised of soldiers. This shift away from funding cancer delegations has reaffirmed the sentiment among many Iraqis that the post-2003 governments have largely ignored the population's cancer burden.

The preceding discussion points to the fact that cancer is a central site for understanding the increased disease burden in Iraq, the unraveling of the country's healthcare apparatus, and the shifting geography of care. The next section examines how cancer patients navigate this geography.[9]

Case Study 1: Financial Burdens on the Kinship Network

I first met Abu Samir[10] and his nephew Abdulrahman in the summer of 2014 during one of their multiple trips back and forth between Iraq and Lebanon for treatments at various Lebanese hospitals. Upon my arrival to their economy Beirut hotel room ($25/night), I sat on the bed as Abu Samir lowered his body next to me. Abdulrahman prepared a bitter sweet drink, joking that the seed that one boils to release the beverage's flavor had a black coloration in Iraq due to the heat. "The brown Lebanese one will do for now," he said. Iraqis seeking cancer care in Beirut manage to approximate certain features from life back home. For example, some companions of patients travel 30 minutes from the medical district to a bakery across town where high-quality Iraqi-style bread can be purchased at a reasonable price.

Two care-seekers from Baghdad, whom Abu Samir had met at the hospital the day before, arrived to wish him well. Abdulrahman welcomed the additional visitors into the small room. Such ephemeral encounters and relations are central to caring for the sick as they travel for medical treatment and care.[11] Abu Samir placed a pillow next to me and demonstrated how I should prop up my body. "I've got another 10 days here," he said. "And I have chemo in the morning." At that point, Abu Samir had made several trips back and forth between his farm north of Baghdad and Lebanon. The family had spent USD$35,000 on his treatment. The Iraq-Lebanon itinerary was not Abu Samir's first option, however. His treatment journey began two years earlier, as he struggled to arrive at a diagnosis in Iraq.

To Baghdad, Kirkuk, and Erbil

Abu Samir's hometown is located one hour north of Baghdad by car. Despite the proximity of large state-run hospitals and private clinics in Baghdad, Abu Samir's three initial trips to the capital city did not yield a convincing diagnosis for the sharp pain in his neck and his nose bleeds. Consequently, he began making multi-hour trips to various private clinics in the northern cities of Kirkuk and Erbil. At this stage in 2013, cancer had not crossed his mind as a possibility. Multiple failed diagnoses obscured an already difficult process. He explained:

> When I got sick, I went to the doctor in Kirkuk a lot, I went to the doctor more than five times. He said you've got some swelling. On my word, I paid 200, 250, 200 [thousand dinars] each time, and I didn't even have the money for that. So I made the trip to Kirkuk until I got tired of it. So I went to the closest place [to our home]. . . . In truth all

I wanted was there to be someone who'd treat me, any doctor. I went to Doctor Friad in Kirkuk, the one who said I had swelling. He said, "Abu Samir you've got swelling, but no problem we'll give you treatment." Twice I went to this doctor, I did an operation, and the operation cost me a million and a half. . . . I mean . . . million and a half dinars. Nothing resulted from it all.

While a fraction of the expenses that Abu Samir would later incur in Beirut, his difficulty putting together the initial payments to the Kirkuk clinic (250,000 dinars, or USD$225) reveals the ambiguity of socioeconomic position in relation to care-seeking. There is an important distinction between personal wealth and the ability to raise funds across a network of kin and neighbors.

Frustrated with the treatment in Kirkuk, Abu Samir eventually decided to go farther north to a doctor in the capital of the semi-autonomous KRG, Erbil. In Erbil he saw a doctor in a private clinic who determined he needed a biopsy, which he had at the government hospital. The biopsy revealed the presence of tumors. He was instructed to go to the tumors division (*qism owram*) at the central government hospital in Erbil. It was January 2014.

It is important to note that ground transportation between Abu Samir's village, Baghdad, Kirkuk, and Erbil would become increasingly untenable after the rise of *daesh* in June 2014 and the subsequent spread of government-supported militias under the banner of Hashd Shaabi. Particularly Sunni residents of the central and northern provinces reduced ground travel for fear of confrontations at militia-controlled checkpoints. Complicating internal movements further, the KRG government would ultimately heighten security and impede entrance through ground borders at the Erbil and Sulaimani crossings. Air travel would become increasingly essential for both internal and foreign travel.

Traveling Abroad

At the government hospital in Erbil, the oncologist advised that, due to a lack of supplies, Abu Samir would have to wait three months before starting treatment.

The doctor told me, "Abu Samir, you're already advanced in the disease. If you go abroad you'll get treatment fast. But he said it'd be . . . eight thousand dollars." But I didn't even have two million dinars!

During the spring of 2014, they gathered funds from family members, friends, and neighbors. Farming was not nearly as profitable in the post-2003 era due to changes in the local irrigation system that devastated grape production. In 2008, Abu Samir discontinued grape farming and focused on tomatoes, eggplant, cabbage, and cucumbers, which were far less lucrative than grapes had been. Across a fifty-five-person family network and neighbors, they were able to amass USD$30,000. They decided to go to Lebanon at the recommendation of a neighbor who had undergone stomach cancer treatment previously. Abu Samir paid $10,000 on the first entry to AUBMC and $7,500 more every twenty-one days. Although flights cost approximately USD$400, he returned to Salah-a-din during the intermediary periods to avoid the more unpredictable accumulation of costs for meals, hotels, and living expenses in Beirut.

Displaced to Erbil

While going back and forth between Iraq and Lebanon during the spring and summer of 2014, the rise of the Islamic State (ISIS) soon gave the government-supported Hashd Shaabi (Popular Mobilization Forces) pretext to take over Yathrib and expel Sunni residents on the accusation of supporting ISIS. In late 2014, Abu Samir, Hussein, and the rest of the fifty-five-person kinship group fled to Erbil. Under new border regulations following the rise of ISIS, they had to enter the Kurdish Region by plane, which represented an enormous expense for such a large family group. Fortunately, upon arrival to Erbil they managed to establish a sharecropping agreement with a Kurdish landowner.

When I visited the new plot of land in Erbil for the first time in August 2015, I asked Abu Samir about medical expenses. He drew a relation between the costs of care in Lebanon and the costs of displacement:

[In Lebanon], if you go to the guy who does radiation he'll tell you how much it'll cost and then I have to go pay before he'll treat you. But if you stay the night in the hospital you pay the deposit and then whatever you're charged over that amount you have to pay when you exit. It's rare you'll ever get anything back. You'll be paying an additional amount. By God we've suffered from this. And back home I had two cars, a house, farming lands upon which I relied for all my production, it's all reliant on the goodness of God. There every season I was making 50 million [dinars] in income. Here if you make 20 million, then you have to cut that in half, 10 to my partner. Then you have five million in expenses, well really it's six million in seeds and chemicals, three each.

Abu Samir moved seamlessly from describing how he has suffered from the accumulative pricing mechanism at Lebanese hospitals to describing the reduced income of farming resulting from displacement to Erbil. Beirut occupied an ambiguous position: It was where Abu Samir could get high-tech treatment quickly, but it was also where the accumulation of unexpected costs mirrored the economic hardships of displacement. When Abu Samir remarked that he formerly earned 50 million dinars (approximately USD$46,000), he was speaking of the gross agricultural income of a large family unit. In Erbil they now earned a fraction of that amount and had higher expenses. Internally displaced persons typically cannot access federal rations for staples such as rice, sugar, and flour, which are dispersed by provincial governments.

Returns

During my most recent visit to the Erbil farm in March 2016, a group of twelve of Abu Samir's family members spent the morning cutting cabbage and stuffing the newly harvested spheres into clear plastic nylon bags. They filled up the entire lorry provided by the Kurdish landowner. Later that day, one of the young men returned from the market to share the news that the sale of the lorry's contents yielded only USD$220. "There's a lot of work and little benefit," remarked Abu Samir. He blamed the influx of agricultural imports from neighboring countries into the Kurdish region for bottoming out the market. While Abu Samir continues to make regular trips to Beirut, there is little consideration of returning to their village north of Baghdad in the near term. Money for subsequent trips to Beirut will have to be gathered from the diminished pool of funds gained from their sharecropping agreement in Erbil.

Case Study 2: Government Sponsorship

As mentioned at the outset, certain hotels in Beirut have capitalized on business from Iraqi Ministry of Health medical delegations. I first stumbled across delegation members at a restaurant immediately adjacent to one such hotel. The owner of the restaurant introduced me to a group of men my age chatting at one of the tables. Each handed over a business card–sized piece of white paper to the waiter and placed their orders. Puzzled by the moneyless transaction, I asked for clarification. One of them pulled out a stack of thirty or so cards. Each card was inscribed with "two people" in big letters across the center as well as the logo of the "American University of Beirut Medical Center" (AUBMC). They were meal vouchers—one for the patient and one for the companion (*murafiq*). I learned that they were part of an IMOH program that funded bone marrow transplants abroad and included room and board. One of these men was a teacher named Kawa who was accompanying his older brother Salim, a soldier. Kawa and Salim's care-seeking journey spanned several years and a wide geography. Participation in the medical delegation figured as an important yet limited part of a longer treatment trajectory.

From Salah-a-din to Erbil and India

Their treatment itinerary began in 2012. Salim's foot was badly injured in a car crash in their hometown of Tuz, a city in the northern part of the Salah-a-din province. Recognizing the superior quality of care in the KRG, Salim's brothers made arrangements for surgery in the autonomous region's capital city, Erbil, roughly three hours from Tuz. As ethnic Kurds with a branch of the family residing in Erbil, entrance into the KRG would not pose an obstacle. But Salim showed few signs of progress following the surgery. When the attempted surgery in Erbil failed, Kawa made arrangements for Salim to travel to Pune, India. "It was there that [doctors] discovered cancer," Kawa related. Salim began chemotherapy for multiple myeloma. Treatment costs in in India reached

USD$10,000 over four sessions of chemo. At Kawa's urging, Salim's doctors communicated with the Hiwa Hospital in Sulaimani, the second largest city in the KRG. Hiwa confirmed the availability of the appropriate medications to continue Salim's treatment.

Erbil and Sulaimani

Upon confirmation from Hiwa, Kawa and Salim returned to Iraq. As they were provided by a state institution, all chemotherapy treatments at Hiwa would be nearly free of charge. Kawa described the payments as "something symbolic (*fad shi ramsi*)": 500 dinars for entrance, and 500 extra for each additional test (approximately USD40 cents). At Hiwa, Salim received a dose of chemotherapy, but hospital supplies of the drug were running low. Consequently Salim's file was transferred to Erbil's Nanakali Cancer Hospital. Salim underwent approximately twenty sessions of chemotherapy at Nanakali Cancer Hospital during 2013. Kawa took turns with his brothers in accompanying Salim on the daylong journeys. They would typically drive three hours from Tuz to Erbil in the morning, undergo an hour of chemotherapy, visit their Erbil relatives, and then return home to Tuz all in a single day.

It was during one of their trips between Tuz and Erbil that they came upon the Ministry of Health's program for treatment abroad.

> We were going to the doctor in Erbil . . . One day a taxi driver told us that his sister and nephew went to India through a program sponsored by the Iraqi Ministry of Health. I said how? What? He said there's a person in our city that knows the deputy Minister of Health. . . . If you communicate with him, he'll speed things up.

Kawa and his brothers followed suit and contacted the man in Tuz identified by the taxi driver. Soon they started receiving communications from the Baghdad-based Ministry of Health requesting documents and reports from their doctor in Erbil. On the basis of communications between the Ministry and the oncologist in Erbil, Salim qualified for the IMOH's new program for administering bone marrow transplants abroad.

Kawa and Salim's efforts to acquire government support were ultimately successful; however, their attempts were not analogous to the well-honed strategies and tactics of claims-making found in ethnographies of highly centralized bureaucratic states (See Petryna 2002). Knowledge of the government program and the crucial contact arose out of a fortuitous conversation with a taxi driver, a fact that highlights the difficulty of gaining access to knowledge under conditions of war and the unraveling of state institutions.

Beirut

After about a month the IMOH notified Kawa and Salim that their case had been designated for the American University of Beirut Medical Center. They would need to come to Baghdad in order to travel to Beirut with a delegation of ten other patients. Upon arrival to Lebanon, the hotel concierge informed them that an administrator from the hospital would contact them shortly to explain the procedure for the bone marrow transplant and recovery period, which would take one hundred days. The hotel, as a subcontractor of the Iraqi Ministry of Health by way of AUBMC, became a satellite extension of the hospital administration. Fully funded by the Iraqi Ministry of Health, Salim underwent a bone marrow transplant at AUBMC and remained in the hospital for twenty-five days. Even as his health recovered over the next three months, Salim rarely left the hotel room other than for meal times. He received frequent visitors, however, in particular an elderly man from Basra who shared Salim's fondness for discussing politics. Walking remained a struggle due to lingering pain in his foot.

One upside of continuing problems with Salim's foot was that it provided a plausible cover: Over the course of two years of treatments, the brothers had still managed to keep Salim's cancer a secret from their parents. Kawa explained the importance of withholding this knowledge in terms of the added pressures on parents in war context. "My mother, she is always worrying about what will happen to us," he said. In the years following the 2003 US-led invasion, Tuz was transformed into a theater of war. Young men like Kawa avoided errands after dark for fear of accusations of violating curfews. The brothers did not want the news of Salim's cancer to add to these worries, and thus they carefully maintained the fiction of undergoing operations in Beirut for Salim's foot. As they struggled for the sake of Salim's life and well-being, they also labored to preserve and attend to a broader web of relations under the stress of war.[12]

Returns

As Salim's treatment period in Beirut came to an end, they returned to Tuz and immediately found themselves in a city besieged by rival militia groups. Over the next few months, Salim's condition continued to improve as he took his cancer drugs. As is often the case, these medications were not available in the state-run hospital and had to be purchased privately in a pharmacy. As Kawa and I drove between Erbil and Sulaimani during the following summer of 2015, he told me: "For us, praise God, we can pay for the medication, but it's still hard. For others, I don't know how they do it." The brothers set up a small window shop that sells soda and snacks where Salim could sit and make a modest income. With recent clashes between the *peshmerga* (Kurdish military forces) and different militias rocking the city, business has generally been slow.

Discussion and Conclusions

Navigating the emerging geography of cancer care involves uncertain movements across clinical sites within and outside of Iraq. For Abu Samir and his family, Lebanon was their third treatment destination after multiple trips to the Iraqi cities of Kirkuk and Erbil. We cannot presume a correlation between personal wealth and the capacity to travel abroad. Abu Samir's fifty-five-person kinship network (three households) were displaced farmers working as sharecroppers. The capacity to raise money for treatment required the combined efforts of three households, in addition to the sales of significant possessions. War-related displacement created added pressures and economic uncertainties for the family network and compromised the sustainability of Abu Samir's treatment itinerary.

Kawa and Salim's story maps out a geography that spanned from their home of Tuz in Salah-a-din, to India, to the northern Iraqi cities of Erbil and Sulaimani, and to Beirut. Government sponsorship was a temporary condition and represented only a small stint within a much longer treatment trajectory. For Kawa and Salim, private and public stints of treatment overlapped. They began with privately funded chemotherapy in India, followed by state oncology in Iraq, followed by state-funded private oncology in Lebanon, and have (for now) culminated with self-funded pharmaceutical purchases due to the absence of the required drug in Iraqi state-run hospitals. It is not surprising that Kawa and Salim did not consider their status to be fundamentally distinct from the self-funded patients they encountered in Beirut: The bone marrow transplant was not the first nor was it the final stop on a much longer treatment journey encompassing various private and public healthcare structures.

These cases highlight that the growing phenomenon of travel between Iraq and neighboring countries for oncology places enormous strains on kinship networks. Earlier anthropological engagements with international therapeutic itineraries have called attention to the massive inequalities that generate care-seeking trajectories across borders in the Middle East and beyond, and the resulting financial burdens placed on families (Kangas 2010; Inhorn and Patrizio 2009); however, these studies have yet to analyze how wars in the region have generated and shaped such trajectories. One significant product of the 2003 invasion and subsequent occupation has been a redistribution of healthcare care-seeking pathways across borders, forcing families and communities to negotiate the financial losses of war while also confronting the additional expenses of private healthcare abroad. While kinship networks enable the cobbling together of resources and information, the highly contingent character of the care-seeking journeys for both privately and publicly funded patients speaks not only to the uncertainties of chronic illness but also the difficulties of navigating healthcare under war conditions. As both cases show, conflict in Iraq has produced violent evictions from homes, transformed household budgets and income generation strategies, and crippled public healthcare institutions.[13]

Understanding the burdens of war on families and communities requires transnational frameworks and methodologies that span a lengthy research period. Illness itineraries are important lenses into transnational processes as they map out assemblages of institutions, relationships, and social spaces across a region. Given the disproportionate amount of media attention devoted to the movement of Syrian and Iraqi migrants into Europe, it is important for anthropologists to understand how individuals and families continuing to reside within the Middle East region have also engaged in survival strategies involving cross-border mobilities. These movements within the region are painfully under-theorized, and thus the paradigmatic scholarly discourses of humanitarianism remain tethered to European frameworks. Cross-border movements in the Middle East go beyond refugee-style migration. The work of dwelling and survival within Iraq increasingly involves transnational strategies. Poor security and the deterioration of crucial infrastructures such as healthcare have generated diverse forms of mobility between Iraq and regional countries, unsettling a picture of living and dying tethered to local relations and institutions. Scholars studying regions transformed by war must explore mobilities that are not oriented around the hopes of leaving and securing citizenship elsewhere, but rather the hopes of remaining and living on.

NOTES

1 Fieldwork for this project is ongoing. I have conducted fieldwork in Beirut over the course of research stints in 2012, 2014, 2015, and 2016, in addition to exploratory visits in Erbil/Sulaimani in 2015 and 2016. I have also visited clinical sites in Amman, Jordan during a one-week visit in 2015. From May 2016 to May 2017, I divided my time between Beirut and Erbil/Sulaimani to complete my work. The research has been supported by the Social Science Research Council.

2 Baghdad remains an enormously important center for care in Iraq, including for oncology. In highlighting these shifts in the geography of care, the point is not to diminish the ongoing role of the capital city in providing care for countless Iraqis.

3 Other terms have been proposed (see Inhorn and Patrizio 2009). My goal in this chapter is not to put forth additional, more refined terms. I have variously used the language of medical "journeys," "itineraries," and "travel." While I agree they are preferable to "tourism," it is also true that even supposedly neutral terms of movement such as "travel" carry problematic connotations of their own (see Clifford 1997).

4 See Skelton 2013 for a more thorough discussion of the politics of evidence surrounding DU.

5 While chemotherapy and radiotherapy are restricted by law to Iraqi state-run hospitals, people often go to private clinics in search of diagnoses or, subsequently, for cancer-related surgeries.

6 Interview, March 5, 2016.

7 This information is based on fieldwork visits to Hiwa Hospital, Zhianawa Cancer Center, and conversations with oncologists and radiologists.
8 Hashd Shaabi is often translated "The Popular Mobilization." It is an umbrella organization encompassing multiple militias arising in response to Ayatollah Sistani's call to combat *daesh* in 2014. See this announcement in Arabic at the Ministry of Health website: "*Al-sayda wazirat al-saha tabhath ma' mudeer al-istiqdam wa al-ikhla' al-tubi irsal jurha al-'amiliyat al-'askariyah*" [The Iraqi Minister of Health Discusses the Sending Abroad of the Wounded from Military Operations with the Director of Recruitment and Medical Evacuations]. Iraqi Ministry of Health, "*Al-sayda wazirat al-saha tabhath ma' mudeer al-istiqdam wa al-ikhla' al-tubi irsal jurha al-'amiliyat al-'askariyah*" [The Iraqi Minister of Health Discusses the Sending Abroad of the Wounded from Military Operations with the Director of Recruitment and Medical Evacuations], 2015, http://www.moh.gov.iq.
9 I will recount the two cases in a linear fashion (Das 2014), but it is important to note that they were shared with me in small fragments over the course of multiple fieldwork stints in Lebanon and Iraq and through two years of frequent phone calls.
10 All names are pseudonyms. Also, readers with a medical background might note a lack of details regarding the specifics of the patient's case from a biomedical standpoint. I have omitted certain specifics for privacy concerns.
11 See also El Moudden 1990 and Dewachi 2015.
12 Here I am thinking of Al Mohammad and Peluso's (2012, 49) discussion of the forms of kindness, care, and attentiveness by which Iraqis have been able to preserve one another and live through the post-invasion era.
13 The data for these cases were collected during a limited period (2014–2016). A continuation of these cases can be found in Skelton (2018).

REFERENCES

Al-Mohammad, H., and D. Peluso. 2012. "Ethics and the 'Rough Ground' of the Everyday: The Overlappings of Life in Post Invasion Iraq." *HAU: Journal of Ethnographic Theory* 2(2): 42–58.

Al-Ta'I, A. 2015. "The Committee for Treatment Outside of Iraq: Mysteries and Secrets Surrounding the Waste of Lives and Money [*Lajnat al-ilaj kharij al-Iraq: khafaya wa asrar 'an hadir lil-arwah wa al-amwaal*]." Al Bayan. Retrieved from http://albayynanew.com.

Anderson, B. 2015. "Beirut Hospital Offers Hope for Civilians Injured in Iraq, Syria." *Wall Street Journal*, June 28.

Appadurai, A. 1996. *Modernity at Large: Cultural Dimensions of Globalization* (Vol. 1). Minneapolis: University of Minnesota Press.

Carrera, P., and J. Bridges. 2006. "Health and Medical Tourism: What They Mean and Imply for Health Care Systems." *Health and Ageing* Volume 15.

Ciment, J. 1998. "Iraq Blames Gulf War Bombing for Increase in Child Cancers." *British Medical Journal* 317(7173): 1612.

Clifford, J. 1997. *Routes: Travel and Translation in the Late Twentieth Century*. Cambridge, MA: Harvard University Press.
Das, V. 2014. *Affliction: Health, Disease, Poverty*. New York: Fordham University Press.
Dewachi, O. 2015. "When Wounds Travel." *Medicine Anthropology Theory* 2(3): 61–82.
Dewachi, O., M. Skelton, V. K. Nguyen, F. M. Fouad, G. A. Sitta, Z. Maasri, and R. Giacaman. 2014. "Changing Therapeutic Geographies of the Iraqi and Syrian Wars." *The Lancet* 383(9915): 449–457.
Diaz, J., and R. Garfield. 2003. "Iraq Health and Nutrition Watching Brief." Geneva: WHO and UNICEF, July.
Duffy, J. 2003. "Iraq's Cancer Children Overlooked in War." *BBC*, April 29. Retrieved from news.bbc.co.uk.
El Moudden, A. 1990. "The Ambivalence of *Rihla*: Community Integration and Self-definition in Moroccan Travel Accounts, 1300–1800." *Muslim Travelers, Migration, and the Religious Imagination*, edited by D. F. Eickelman and J. Piscatori, 69–84. Berkeley: University of California Press.
Even-Paz, Z., and J. Shani. 1989. "The Dead Sea and Psoriasis." *International Journal of Dermatology* 28(1): 1–9.
Garfield, R., S. Zaidi, and J. Lennock. 1997. "Medical Care in Iraq after Six Years of Sanctions." *BMJ* 315(7120): 1474–1475.
Inhorn, M. C. 2011. "Globalization and Gametes: Reproductive 'Tourism,' Islamic Bioethics, and Middle Eastern Modernity." *Anthropology and Medicine* 18(1): 87–103.
Inhorn, M. C., and P. Patrizio. 2009. "Rethinking Reproductive 'Tourism' as Reproductive 'Exile.'" *Fertility and Sterility* 92(3): 904–906.
Iraqi Ministry of Health. 2014. Ministerial Order of the High Committee for the Treatment of Patients Outside of Iraq. Issued by Ayman 'Asim Muhammad Ameen on March 2.
Kangas, B. 2010. "Traveling for Medical Care in a Global World." *Medical Anthropology* 29(4): 344–362.
Kevan, S. M. 1993. "Quests for Cures: A History of Tourism for Climate and Health." *International Journal of Biometeorology* 37(3): 113–124.
MedAct. 2008. *Rehabilitation Under Fire: Health Care in Iraq, 2003–2007*. London: MedAct.
Middle East Health. 2013. "Lebanon's Leading Hospitals Continue to Attract Foreign Patients." *Middle East Health Magazine*, July 18.
Mula-Hussain, L. 2010. "The Challenges of Providing Cancer Care in a War-torn Nation." *American Society of Clinical Oncology Connection*, August 10.
Mula-Hussain, L. 2012. *Cancer Care in Iraq: A Descriptive Study*. Saarbrucken: Lampert Academic.
Niv, A. 1989. "Health Tourism in Israel: A Developing Industry." *Tourist Review* 44(4): 30–32.
Parkinson, S. E., and O. Behrouzan. 2015. "Negotiating Health and Life: Syrian Refugees and the Politics of Access in Lebanon." *Social Science and Medicine* 146: 324–331.

Peterson, S. 2000. "Depleted Uranium Haunts Kosovo and Iraq." *Middle East Report* 215 (Summer): 14–15.

Petryna, A. 2002. *Life Exposed: Biological Citizens after Chernobyl*. Princeton, NJ: Princeton University Press.

Ramírez de Arellano, A. B. 2007. "Patients without Borders: The Emergence of Medical Tourism." *International Journal of Health Services 37*(1): 193–198.

Sikora, K. 1999. "Cancer Services Are Suffering in Iraq." *British Medical Journal 318*(7177): 203–204.

Skelton, M. 2013. "Health and Health Care Decline in Iraq: The Example of Cancer and Oncology." Retrieved from http://watson.brown.edu/costsofwar.

Skelton, M. 2018. "Cancer Itineraries Across Borders in Post-invasion Iraq: War, Displacement, and Geographies of Care." PhD diss., Johns Hopkins University.

8

War and Its Consequences for Cancer Trends and Services in Iraq

LAYTH MULA-HUSSAIN

Iraq is a Middle Eastern, multiethnic, developing country, with an estimated population of around 37 million people, living in nineteen governorates.[1] This historically prosperous land, with a rich ancient heritage, has seen all its living systems, including its cancer care services system, decimated by wars, sanctions, and embargo over the last quarter of a century and in particular, from August 1990 until today.

Cancer trends and care in Iraq have transformed as a result. Wars, sanctions, and embargo have affected the types of cancer that Iraqis get, the stages at which cancers are diagnosed, the care facilities available to cancer patients, and human resources in oncology. With reduced services, cancers are discovered in more advanced stages, reducing curability, and patients' suffering has increased.

Iraq, Health, and Cancer

In a country where leaving one's house each day can be deadly, cancer may seem a minor concern. But it can, of course, be as potentially fatal. Iraq has seen an increase in its cancer rate, and at the same time, a reduction in the human and material resources needed to fight this disease.

The story of Iraq's experience with war has many chapters, but the most consequential began in August 1990 with the implementation of the United Nations sanctions and trade embargo; continued through the 1991 US-led invasion to expel the Iraqi military from Kuwait; through the US-led invasion in 2003 to unseat Saddam Hussein and the long US occupation; through the takeover by the Islamic State of Iraq and the

Levant (ISIL) of parts of the country; and through the Western nations' military campaign to destroy this terrorist group. Wars, the sanctions, and the embargo decimated all of Iraq's living systems—including its cancer care system.

Iraq was once quite developed and prosperous, and the health status of Iraqis was excellent in comparison with neighboring countries in the Middle East. The Iraqi Ministry of Health (MOH) was established in 1920, and the first modern medical school, the Iraqi Royal Medical College, was established in the capital, Baghdad, in 1927. The population's health status was steadily improving after these landmark dates until 1990. During this period, infant mortality fell by about two-thirds (from 117 to 40 deaths per 1,000 births) and child mortality fell by 70 percent (from 171 to 50 deaths per 1,000 births). The health system developed well in this era and focused on a highly centralized, hospital-based, capital-intensive model of curative care. It was fully subsidized, with free healthcare provided to all Iraqis. Many patients from neighboring countries used to seek care in Baghdad health facilities with their highly trained physicians.

By the late 1990s, health indicators began to decline. Life expectancies in Iraq, which had been rapidly rising during the 1960s, '70s, and '80s across all of Iraq's Middle Eastern neighbors except for Yemen, began to fall.[2] Shortages of food and medicines limited access to essential goods for the majority of the population. The food rations provided by the Iraqi government met only part of the population's food needs. Many hospitals and health centers were damaged during the invasions of 1991 and 2003 and the ensuing wars. A good number of medical personnel left the country, and financial resources for the health sector declined precipitously. The supply of electricity became erratic, making many health facilities nonfunctional or ineffective. Health sector imports (particularly medicines and medical equipment) had fallen from US$500 million in 1989 to US$50 million in 1991. Overall health spending per capita fell from a minimum of US$86 to US$17 in 1996. The capacity of the curative health system was, by the late 1990s, greatly reduced (Alwan 2004; Sen 2003).

Cancer is not a single disease like diabetes mellitus, for example, but rather a group of diseases that can develop in many body tissues, and it is characterized by an uncontrolled growth and spread of abnormal cells (American Cancer Society 2011). It is a leading cause of death globally and its burden has more than doubled during the past thirty years worldwide, due both to longer life spans and to lifestyle and environmental issues, including smoking, obesity, and sedentarism. In 2012, it was estimated that cancer had claimed more than 14 million new patients, 8 million deaths, and 32 million five-year survivors (Stewart and Wild 2014). By 2030, there could be 27 million new patients, 17 million cancer deaths, and 75 million survivors (Boyle and Levin 2009).

Cancer care and cancer control are therefore becoming ever more integral or significant components in any healthcare system. Cancer care is the active treatment and follow-up of the cancer as a disease, while cancer control is the larger umbrella that describes the totality of activities and interventions intended to reduce the burden of cancer in a population, either by reducing cancer incidence or mortality, or by alleviating the suffering of people with cancer (Sloan and Gelband 2007).

Over the last quarter of a century, cancer incidence rates are reported to be increasing in Iraq, likely accounted for variously by war pollutants such as Depleted Uranium; by the deterioration of medical awareness; by overall low socioeconomic status; and by denial of, or cultural misperceptions about, cancer. The increase in reported cancer cases may also be due to improvement in the cancer registration system to some extent. Between 50 percent and 80 percent of cancers in Iraq are detected at advanced stages of the disease and are thus incurable even if the best therapies were to be offered. Patients with potentially curable cancers can only receive drugs locally available at the time of their treatment (Busby, Hamdan, and Ariabi 2010; Deli and Ibrahim 2005; Sen 2003). In ideal circumstances, three lines of cytotoxic drugs would be available, each composed of one to five drugs. The oncologist would normally begin treatment with the first line and its full components before moving to the second and third lines. However, in Iraq, due to shortages of many drugs, physicians are giving what is available and not necessarily what should be given. Obviously, this can damage therapeutic outcomes.

Karol Sikora, the chief at the World Health Organization's cancer program, reported the following observation after a visit to Iraq in 1999:

> It was immediately clear that there were staggering deficiencies in cancer treatment facilities because of the United Nations sanctions, which are

intended to exclude food and medicines. A cancer centre without a single analgesic; a radiotherapy unit where each patient needs one hour under the machine because the radiation source is so old; and children dying of curable cancers because drugs run out are all accepted as normal. . . . Somehow cancer care has become a Cinderella service. Requested radiotherapy equipment, chemotherapy drugs, and analgesics are consistently blocked by United States and British advisers. There seems to be a rather ludicrous notion that such agents could be converted into chemical or other weapons. . . . Whatever the political legitimacy of the embargo, the needless suffering of those with cancer is an unacceptable outcome. (Sikora 1999)

After the 2003 invasion, volatile security conditions in most parts of Iraq led to a number of deleterious consequences for the country's health sector. Those included the outflow of remaining Iraqi scientists and medical experts; slow progress toward the rehabilitation of the health sector; and reallocation of government financial resources from civil and developmental sectors such as the health sector, for example, to the security sector.

I now move on to present more details on cancer trends and health services in this war-torn country from the last twenty-five years.

Cancer Trends

The official Iraqi Cancer Registry (ICR), the nineteenth edition of which was released in late 2015, reflects cancer data for 2012. In that year, the Iraqi population was estimated to be 32,489,972 and there were 21,101 reported cancer cases (tables 8.1 and 8.2). A total of 10,278 cancer-related deaths were reported, of which 5,346 took place among males and 4,932 among females (table 8.3). No information was available about the presenting stage at diagnosis (Iraqi Cancer Registry Center 2015).

When we examine the crude incidence rates in the Iraqi governorates, we see that it ranged from 24.31 to 85.41 per 100,000 population, with a mean of 61.69 (figure 8.1). If we compare this mean figure (61.69) in 2012 with the one from twenty years ago, in 1992, we see a strong increase from 44.99 (figure 8.2). In this regard, one can ask: Why is there such a wide range of incidence during the period from 1992 through

TABLE 8.1. The top ten cancers in Iraqi males in 2012 (2012 ICR)

Primary Site	Number of Cases	% of Total	Registered Cases/10⁵ Pop.
1—Bronchus and Lung	1,326	14.28	7.61
2—Leukemia	847	9.12	4.86
3—Urinary Bladder	843	9.08	4.84
4—Non-Hodgkin's Lymphoma	695	7.48	3.99
5—Colorectal Cancer	621	6.69	3.56
6—Brain and Other CNS	567	6.04	3.22
7—Prostate	421	4.53	2.42
8—Stomach	417	4.49	2.39
9—Skin	361	3.89	2.07
10—Larynx	305	3.28	1.75
Total Ten	6,403	68.89	36.72
All Sites	9,268	100.00	53.31

Estimated Male Population in Iraq 2012: (17,419,724).

TABLE 8.2. The top ten cancers in Iraqi females in 2012 (2012 ICR)

Primary Site	Number of Cases	% of Total	Registered Cases/10⁵ Pop.
1—Breast	4,024	33.95	23.97
2—Leukemia	683	5.76	4.07
3—Brain and Other CNS	584	4.93	3.48
4—Colorectal Cancer	545	4.60	3.25
5—Non-Hodgkin's Lymphoma	541	4.57	3.22
6—Ovary	519	4.38	3.09
7—Bronchus and Lung	516	4.35	3.07
8—Thyroid Gland	446	3.76	2.66
9—Stomach	320	2.70	1.91
10—Skin	316	2.67	1.88
Total Ten	8,494	71.83	50.60
All Sites	11,851	100.00	70.59

Estimated Female Population in Iraq 2012: (16,787,524).

2012 and among different Iraqi governorates? What are the possible explanations for these differences? Actually, these reported rates in the last years have been highlighted as an increase in incidence by some of the investigators in this period of time (Busby et al. 2010; Deli and Ibrahim 2005; Habib et al. 2007; Hagopian et al. 2010).

In this 2012 registry, the top ten cancers in Iraqi males were cancers of the lungs, blood, urinary bladder, non-Hodgkin's lymphoma, colorectal, central nervous system (CNS), prostate, stomach, skin, and larynx (table 8.1). The top ten cancers in Iraqi females were cancers of the breast, blood, CNS, colorectal, non-Hodgkin's lymphoma, lung, ovary, thyroid, skin, and urinary bladder (table 8.2). The top ten cancers in children (0–14 years old) were leukemia, brain tumors, Non-Hodgkin's lymphoma, Hodgkin's lymphoma, kidney tumors, bone tumors, eye tumors, soft tissue tumors, ovarian tumors, and adrenal gland tumors (Iraqi Cancer Registry Center 2015). If we come back to the top ten in different years, in all Iraqis (males and females), we can see that CNS tumors ranked eighth in 1998 (Iraqi Cancer Registry Center 2006a), fourth in 2004 (Iraqi Cancer Registry Center 2006b), third in 2009 (Iraqi Cancer Registry Center 2012), and then sixth in 2012 (Iraqi Cancer Registry Center 2015). While leukemia ranked fifth in 1998 (Iraqi Cancer Registry Center 2006a), second in 2004 (Iraqi Cancer Registry Center 2006b), fifth in

TABLE 8.3. The top ten fatal cancers in Iraqis in 2012 (2012 ICR)

Site	Total	Male	Female	Percentage	Incidence Rate
Bronchus and Lung	1,756	1,270	486	17.09	5.13
Brain	1,122	576	546	10.92	3.28
Breast	1,008	0	1,008	9.81	2.95
Leukemia	994	525	469	9.67	2.91
Liver	673	333	340	6.55	1.97
Stomach	539	303	236	5.24	1.58
Urinary Bladder	536	395	141	5.22	1.57
Colorectal	504	280	224	4.90	1.47
Pancreas	472	268	204	4.59	1.38
Lymph Nodes (Lymphoma)	361	202	159	3.51	1.06
Total Ten	7,965	4,152	3,813	77.50	23.28
All Cancer Deaths	10,278	5,346	4,932	100.00	30.05

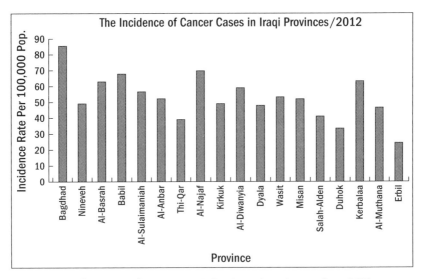

Figure 8.1. Incidence rate of cancer cases in Iraqi provinces in 2012 (2012 ICR)

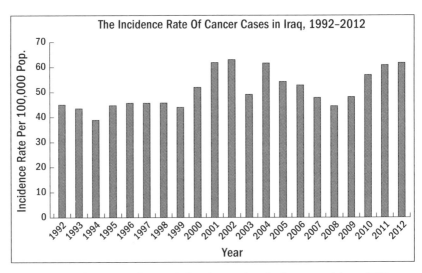

Figure 8.2. Incidence rate of cancer in Iraq in two decades (1992–2012) (2012 ICR)

2009 (Iraqi Cancer Registry Center 2012), and then third in 2012 (Iraqi Cancer Registry Center 2015). Tables 8.4 and 8.5 show the top ten cancers in Iraq from the 2012 ICR in comparison with the top ten cancers in three neighboring countries (Jordan, Kuwait, and Iran) and three non-neighboring countries (Japan, Germany, and United States) from the

2012 GLOBOCAN (age 15 and over) (Ferlay et al. 2013) for males and females. Clearly, there are important differences between the top ten cancers in Iraq and the top ten cancers in these six countries. What explains these differences? And why, in particular, are leukemia and CNS tumors on the rise in Iraq?

TABLE 8.4. Top ten cancers in Iraqi males (2012 ICR) compared to the top ten in six countries (2012 GLOBOCAN)

Iraq	Jordan	Kuwait	Iran	USA	Germany	Japan
Lung	CRC	Prostate	Stomach	Prostate	Prostate	Stomach
Leukemia	Lung	CRC	Bladder	Lung	CRC	CRC
Bladder	Prostate	Lung	Prostate	CRC	Lung	Lung
NHL	Bladder	NHL	CRC	Bladder	Bladder	Prostate
CRC	*Leukemia*	Bladder	Lung	CMM	Kidney	Liver
CNS	Stomach	*Leukemia*	Esophagus	Kidney	CMM	Esophagus
Prostate	Larynx	Liver	*Leukemia*	NHL	Stomach	Pancreas
Stomach	NHL	Pancreas	NHL	*Leukemia*	*Leukemia*	Bladder
Skin	Liver	Stomach	*CNS*	Liver	NHL	NHL
Larynx	Pancreas	Kidney	Larynx	Pancreas	Testis	Kidney

Abbreviations: Central Nervous System (CNS), Colo-Rectal Cancers (CRC), Cutaneous Malignant Melanoma (CMM), Hodgkin's Lymphoma (HL), Non-Hodgkin's Lymphoma (NHL).

TABLE 8.5. Top ten cancers in Iraqi females (2012 ICR) compared to the top ten in six countries (2012 GLOBOCAN)

Iraq	Jordan	Kuwait	Iran	USA	Germany	Japan
Breast	Breast	Breast	Breast	Breast	Breast	Breast
Leukemia	CRC	CRC	CRC	Lung	CRC	CRC
CNS	Thyroid	Corpus Ut	Stomach	CRC	Lung	Stomach
CRC	NHL	Thyroid	Esophagus	Thyroid	CMM	Lung
NHL	Ovary	*Leukemia*	Lung	Corpus Ut	Corpus Ut	Cervix Ut
Ovary	Stomach	Lung	Ovary	CMM	Cervix Ut	Corpus Ut
Lung	Corpus Ut	Ovary	*Leukemia*	NHL	Kidney	Ovary
Thyroid	*Leukemia*	Cervix Ut	Thyroid	Kidney	Ovary	Pancreas
Stomach	Lung	NHL	*CNS*	Ovary	NHL	Thyroid
Skin	Pancreas	Bladder	NHL	*Leukemia*	Pancreas	NHL

Abbreviations: Central Nervous System (CNS), Colo-Rectal Cancers (CRC), Cutaneous Malignant Melanoma (CMM), Hodgkin's Lymphoma (HL), Non-Hodgkin's Lymphoma (NHL), Uteri (Ut).

TABLE 8.6. Number and incidence rates in males and females during the period 1992–2012

Years	No. of New Cases Registered	Male		Female		Registered Cases / 10^5 Pop.
		No.	%	No.	%	
1992	8,562	4,735	55.54	3,791	44.46	44.99
1993	8,471	4,632	54.68	3,839	45.32	43.49
1994	7,785	4,230	54.34	3,555	45.66	38.91
1995	7,948	4,344	54.66	3,604	45.34	44.69
1996	8,360	4,466	53.42	3,894	46.58	45.69
1997	8,592	4,521	52.62	4,071	47.38	45.67
1998	9,033	4,774	52.85	4,259	47.15	45.74
1999	8,936	4,556	50.98	4,380	49.02	43.95
2000	10,888	5,376	49.38	5,512	50.63	52.00
2001	13,332	6,758	50.69	6,574	49.31	61.83
2002	13,985	6,964	49.80	7,021	50.20	62.97
2003	11,248	5,698	50.66	5,550	49.34	49.17
2004	14,520	7,525	51.83	6,995	48.17	61.63
2005	15,172	7,505	49.47	7,667	50.53	54.26
2006	15,226	7,377	48.45	7,849	51.54	52.84
2007	14,213	6,656	46.83	7,557	53.16	47.88
2008	14,180	6,589	46.47	7,591	53.53	44.46
2009	15,251	7,201	47.22	8,050	52.78	48.16
2010	18,482	8,544	46.23	9,938	53.77	56.89
2011	20,278	9,352	46.12	10,926	53.88	60.82
2012	21,101	9,268	43.92	11,833	56.08	61.69
Total	265,527	134,196	49.36	134,456	50.64	—

From 1992 to 1994, and from 2005 to 2012, Kurdistan Region included.
From 1995 to 2004, Kurdistan Region not included.

In my view, the relative rise in these two cancers can be attributed to the environmental hazards associated with warfare. There is strong evidence linking exposure to ionizing radiation and development of brain cancer and/or leukemia. Citing a series of studies on nuclear workers in the United States between 1950 through the 1990s, the Center for Environmental Health Studies states that there is a significant association between exposure to ionizing radiation, on the one hand, and the incidence of brain cancer deaths and nervous system tumors, on the other.[3] Another paper by the Center found a strong association between exposure to ionizing radiation among US nuclear workers and deaths from leukemia.[4] According to the World Health Organization, "retention of any radioactive material in the body will have associated an increase in the probability of cancer," though the increase is small and depends on the amount of radiation dose (World Health Organization 2001). In the Gulf Wars, the United States and the UK made extensive use of depleted uranium weapons, which are weakly radioactive. That said, more research is needed on whether there exists a causal relationship between use of depleted uranium weapons in the Gulf Wars and increased risk of cancer among Iraqi civilians (Marshall 2008).

Another interesting cancer trend is the rise of cancers in females (as in table 8.6) which were once less frequent in comparison to males in Iraq (44% versus 55.5%) in 1992. After that year, the frequency in females gradually increased and their rate became equivalent to that of males in 2000; in the last several years, cancers in females have surpassed males in frequency (56% versus 44%), as is obvious in 2012 (Iraqi Cancer Registry Center 2015). It is important to work toward a research-based understanding of what is behind these trends in cancer in Iraq (Mula-Hussain 2015).

Cancer Care Services

There are striking deficiencies in all aspects of cancer care services, not only in the small cities, but in the major ones as well. Although we have chemotherapy and some radiotherapy services in major Iraqi cities, there are no recognized surgical oncology services and very few palliative care services. In addition, Iraq does not have an academic comprehensive cancer center, a type of medical facility that is known to improve cancer care outcomes, in addition to advancing knowledge and training among local health professionals (Mula-Hussain 2010).

Government Regulation No. 15 was issued in 2002 by the Ministry of Health in Baghdad. It was to establish the first comprehensive cancer center (Saddam Center for the Diagnosis, Treatment and Research of Tumors) based in Baghdad. This center was planned to provide medical, research, and training services in this field and to keep abreast of scientific developments that occur inside and outside Iraq. It was going to be composed of departments of surgical oncology, diagnostic oncology, nuclear medicine (with a cyclotron for producing radioactive materials), radiation oncology, medical adult and pediatric oncology, clinical pathology and bone marrow transplant, tumor pathology, tumor biology, rehabilitation medicine, and the department of medical statistics and oncological epidemiology, and a focus on early detection, health education, and cancer prevention, and the department for "anesthesia, pain treatment and palliative care." Unfortunately, with the invasion and occupation the followed in 2003, this project came to a halt (Mula-Hussain 2012).

The Annual Report of the MOH in 2010 (Ministry of Health 2011) puts the available number of physicians in Iraq at 24,750 (around 750 physicians per million population). Of those, only thirty-one were cancer physicians/oncologists (around 1 per million population). This constitutes a severe shortage of cancer physicians among the total number of physicians in Iraq. Comparing this rate (1 per million) in Iraq with the international recommendations on consultant staffing of 8–12 cancer physicians per million population (Expert Working Group on Radiation Oncology Services 2003), we can see how far Iraq must go to improve its situation, with an average of 320 +/−30 more oncologists needed in the country.

The five-year plan of the Iraqi National Cancer Control Program (INCCP for 2010–2014) that was endorsed by the Iraqi Cancer Board (ICB) at the MOH in 2010 presented an excellent plan to improve cancer control in Iraq, including improvements in cancer prevention, early detection, diagnosis, and treatment as well as in palliative care (Ministry of Health 2010). This program has been associated with some achievements (such as the passage of a tobacco control law in early 2012) and some disappointments (such as in the lack of development of radiotherapy facilities). In the latter, the INCCP stated that there were six functioning linear accelerators (machines used for radiotherapy) as of February 2010 in four Iraqi cities (three in Baghdad, one in Mosul, one in Sulaymaniyah, and one in Erbil). The INCCP called attention to an urgent need in two years (2010–2011) for an additional fifteen machines to be distributed in eight cities (i.e., for a total of twenty-one functioning machines in eight Iraqi cities) and another ten machines in the following three years (2012–2014) for the remaining ten governorates (which constitutes a total of thirty-one machines in the entire country by the end of the INCCP in 2014). Yet 2011 concluded without any additional radiotherapy equipment. As of April 2018, only ten functioning machines were added to the previously mentioned ones. This meant a total of sixteen functioning machines were available in seven Iraqi cities (five in Baghdad, three in Basra, two in Sulaymaniyah, two in Babil, two in Misan, one in Erbil, one in Najaf, while the one in Mosul became nonfunctioning during the ISIS occupation of the city).

Finally, one can add that the financial resources that MOH has allocated for all of the country's healthcare needs are inadequate. There is a striking difference between the governmental allocation for the health sector in 2010 in Iraq (that is IQD 6,547.75 billion or approximately US$5.45 billion in total, and US$168 per person) and that in Canada, for example, whose population is quite similar in size to that of Iraq (approximately CA$191.6 billion in total and CA$5,614 per person) (Canadian Institute for Health Information 2010; Ministry of Health 2011).[5]

In summary, cancer care services in Iraq have been negatively affected in the last twenty-five years due to wars, embargo, sanctions, occupation, corruption, and rampant insecurity. Accordingly, the current condition of the Iraqi healthcare system is far below international standards. Iraq has:

- Suboptimal cancer care facilities (including radiotherapy, chemotherapy, cancer surgery, and palliative care facilities; as well as suboptimal bone marrow transplant capacity, among other forms of cancer care).
- No comprehensive academic cancer center.
- Suboptimal cancer research in Iraq, possibly related to inadequate funding, lack of capacity to host interested scientists, lack of time, and difficult life circumstances of scholars, among other factors.
- Suboptimal human resources and training programs for cancer care (Mula-Hussain 2014).[6]
- Slow achievement of the required improvements in cancer care in Iraq.
- Suboptimal governmental financial resources for the health sector in general, in addition to the absence or inadequacy of the non-governmental sector (for profit or not-for-profit) in cancer care in Iraq.

Conclusion

Cancer care services in Iraq have been negatively affected over the past twenty-five years, though a close examination of cancer trends across different Iraqi governorates reveals a complex picture. To reach sound conclusions about the extent and determinants of cancer trends in Iraq, immense multi-spectrum, analytic efforts are needed. Both local and international experts should pay attention to these cancer trends (in order to deepen their understanding) and to the available services (in order to tailor the required services accordingly).

As the case of cancer trends and care in Iraq shows, war, sanctions, and embargo have far-reaching effects on people's health, including and well beyond injuries, deaths, and illnesses sustained on battlefields. Yet, in spite of the difficult challenges the Iraqi people face, there has been some gradual partial improvement in the health sector in general and the cancer services field in particular from 2009 onward. In order to truly reach the necessary standards of medical care, I suggest the following improvements (Mula-Hussain 2012).

- Policymakers in Iraq should draw up a set of priority areas for decision-making on a comprehensive cancer control program at the national level with a time line. An annual conference and an external audit of the plans and achievements of the ICB and the INCCP should take place.
- A comprehensive academic cancer center staffed by scientist-clinicians in all cancer care specialties is urgently needed. The center would lead nationally coordinated, collaborative, priority-driven, clinical- and laboratory-based research efforts, to better understand cancer trends and risk factors in Iraq.
- Investment by the MOH and the Ministry of Higher Education and Scientific Research should be made to build competent and highly qualified human resources in all specialties of cancer care through sponsored governmental scholarships abroad and suitable incentives and support to encourage the expatriate Iraqi scientists to return to serve in Iraq.
- Sustained commitment at the highest levels of central and local governments is required for cancer care improvement. An example of such commitment would be passage of the first ever cancer control law in Iraq. Actually, the passage of the National Cancer Act of 1971 in the United

States led to many improvements in this regard. That act mandates federal budgetary allocations specifically for cancer prevention, treatment, and research, including for the acquisition of all necessary chemical compounds and other materials required for this research. It precipitated dramatic improvements in cancer outcomes in the decades following its passage.[7]

- Not-for-profit activities and projects delivered by public groups and organizations should be championed by the authorities, to support cancer prevention and care in this war-torn country.

NOTES

1 Estimates of Iraq's population are inadequate given the lack of a census and massive population movements into and out of the country. One 2016 estimate puts the population at 39.3 million people (Worldometers, "Iraq Population," 2018).
2 World Bank, "World Development Indicators 2013," 2016. Life expectancy at birth was estimated, according to the UNDP Human Development Report 2001, to be 59.2 years for males and 62.3 years for females at that time. The only set of figures available at the Ministry of Planning and Development Corporation of Iraq (MOPDC) are for the year 1997: They show a life expectancy of 58 years for males and 59 for females.
3 Center for Environmental Health Studies, "Brain Cancer and Exposure to Ionizing Radiation."
4 Center for Environmental Health Studies, "Leukemia and Exposure to Ionizing Radiation."
5 To put these monetary comparisons in perspective, before 1991, each Iraqi dinar was exchanged in the government banks for about 3.3 US dollars. After the embargo and resulting inflation, each US dollar became equivalent to 2,000–3,000 dinars (down in the last decade to about 1,200–1,300 dinars per dollar). Significant corruption also erodes the amount of healthcare provided per dinar.
6 While Iraq has some services in surgical oncology, radiation oncology, and medical adult/pediatric oncology, there are no surgical oncology training programs in the country. There are two levels of training available in radiation oncology: one two-year program, launched in the 1980s in Baghdad; and a four-year program launched in 2013 in Sulaymaniyah. In medical oncology, there is a three-year pediatric oncology program launched during the 2000s in Baghdad. The adult oncology program was launched in Baghdad in 2012 and in Erbil in 2014.
7 Recognizing the 40th Anniversary of the National Cancer Act of 1971—31 Jan 2012, 112th Congress—2nd Session, 2012).

REFERENCES

Alwan, Aládin. 2004. *Health in Iraq: The Current Situation, Our Vision for the Future and Areas of Work*. 2nd ed. Baghdad: Ministry of Health.

American Cancer Society. 2011. *Global Cancer Facts and Figures 2nd edition*. Atlanta, GA: American Cancer Society. Retrieved from www.cancer.org.

Boyle, Peter, and Bernard Levin. 2009. *World Cancer Report 2008*. Geneva: World Health Organization.

Busby, Chris, Malak Hamdan, and Entesar Ariabi. 2010. "Cancer, Infant Mortality and Birth Sex-Ratio in Fallujah, Iraq 2005–2009." *International Journal of Environmental Research and Public Health* 7 (7): 2828–37. doi:10.3390/ijerph7072828.

Canadian Institute for Health Information. 2010. "Health Care Spending to Reach $192 Billion This Year." *CIHI*, October 28. Retrieved from www.cihi.ca.

Center for Environmental Health Studies. N.d. "Brain Cancer and Exposure to Ionizing Radiation." The MTA Fund Collection at the Kasperson Library, Clark University. Retrieved from www2.clarku.edu/mtafund.

Center for Environmental Health Studies. N.d. "Leukemia and Exposure to Ionizing Radiation." The MTA Fund Collection at the Kasperson Library, Clark University. Retrieved from www2.clarku.edu/mtafund.

Deli, A., and L. Ibrahim. 2005. "Oncology in Iraq." *ASCO News*, 38.

Expert Working Group on Radiation Oncology Services. 2003. *The Development of Radiation Oncology Services in Ireland*. Dublin: Ministry for Health and Children. Retrieved from www.hse.ie.

Ferlay, J., I. Soerjomataram, M. Ervik, R. Dikshit, S. Eser, C. Mathers, M. Rebelo, D. M. Parkin, D. Forman, and F. Bray. 2013. *GLOBOCAN 2012 v1.0, Cancer Incidence and Mortality Worldwide: IARC CancerBase no. 11 [Internet]*. Lyon, France: International Agency for Research on Cancer. Retrieved from http://globocan.iarc.fr.

Habib, Omran S., Jawad K. Al-Ali, Mohammed K. Al-Wiswasi, Narjis A. H. Ajeel, Osama G. Al-Asady, Asaad A. A. Khalaf, and Abbas Z. M. Al-Mayah. 2007. "Cancer Registration in Basrah 2005: Preliminary Results." *Asian Pacific Journal of Cancer Prevention: APJCP* 8 (2): 187–90.

Hagopian, Amy, Riyadh Lafta, Jenan Hassan, Scott Davis, Dana Mirick, and Tim Takaro. 2010. "Trends in Childhood Leukemia in Basrah, Iraq, 1993–2007." *American Journal of Public Health* 100 (6): 1081–87. doi:10.2105/AJPH.2009.164236.

Iraqi Cancer Registry Center. 2006a. *1998–1999 Results of Iraqi Cancer Registry*. Baghdad: Iraqi Cancer Board—Ministry of Health.

Iraqi Cancer Registry Center. 2006b. *2004 Results of Iraqi Cancer Registry*. Baghdad: Iraqi Cancer Board—Ministry of Health.

Iraqi Cancer Registry Center. 2012. *2009 Results of Iraqi Cancer Registry*. 16th ed. Baghdad: Iraqi Cancer Board—Ministry of Health.

Iraqi Cancer Registry Center. 2015. *2012 Results of Iraqi Cancer Registry*. Baghdad: Iraqi Cancer Board—Ministry of Health.

Marshall, Albert C. 2008. "Gulf War Depleted Uranium Risks." *Journal of Exposure Science and Environmental Epidemiology* 18: 95–108. doi: 10.1038/sj.jes.7500551.

Ministry of Health. 2010. *Iraqi National Cancer Control Program (Five Year Plan 2010–2014)*. 2nd ed. Baghdad: Iraqi Cancer Board—Ministry of Health.

Ministry of Health. 2011. *Annual Report for 2010*. Baghdad: Ministry of Health. Retrieved from www.moh.gov.iq.

Mula-Hussain, Layth. 2010. "The Challenges of Providing Cancer Care in a War-torn Nation—The Iraqi Experience." *ASCO Daily News: The Official Daily Newspaper of the American Society of Clinical Oncology (ASCO) Annual Meeting*, June 5.

Mula-Hussain, Layth. 2012. *Cancer Care in Iraq: A Descriptive Study*. 1st ed. Saarbrucken, Germany: LAP Lambert Academic Publishing.

Mula-Hussain, Layth. 2014. "Cancer in Iraq: The Dilemma Continues." *ASCO Daily News: The Official Daily Newspaper of the American Society of Clinical Oncology (ASCO) Annual Meeting*, May 31. Retrieved from http://am.asco.org.

Mula-Hussain, Layth. 2015. "Cancer in a War-torn Arab Community—Iraq: Description of Its Trends." *ACCESS Health Journal* Fall (3).

Sen, Biswajit. 2003. *Iraq Watching Briefs (Health and Nutrition)*. UNICEF. Retrieved from www.unicef.org/evaldatabase.

Sikora, Karol. 1999. "Cancer Services Are Suffering in Iraq." *BMJ* 318 (7177): 203.

Sloan, Frank A., and Hellen Gelband. 2007. *Cancer Control Opportunities in Low- and Middle-Income Countries*. Washington, DC: Institute of Medicine—National Academies Press.

Stewart, B. W., and C. P. Wild, eds. 2014. *World Cancer Report 2014*. Lyon: International Agency for Research on Cancer and World Health Organization.

World Bank. 2016. "World Development Indicators 2013." Retrieved from http://www.indexmundi.com.

World Health Organization. 2001. "Depleted Uranium: Sources, Exposure and Health Effects." Retrieved from http://apps.who.int.

Worldometers. 2018. "Iraq Population." Retrieved from www.worldometers.info.

PART III

United States

9

Imagining Military Suicide

KEN MACLEISH

Military suicide is widely regarded as a crisis in the contemporary United States, and available data seem to bear this out. While the suicide rate among US military personnel has historically been quite low—lower than that among civilians[1]—it began to climb shortly after the beginning of the wars in Iraq and Afghanistan, eventually exceeding the civilian rate, spiking in 2012, and then plateauing after a slight decline. Suicide has for a number of years now been one of the leading causes of death among American military personnel—significantly deadlier than combat, especially now that US ground forces' fighting in Iraq and Afghanistan has largely subsided. With this rise, suicide has increasingly dominated Americans' collective ideas about how war affects the people who are asked to fight it. Military leaders, politicians and policymakers, and the civilian public all regard suicide among service members as a scandal, a sudden and anomalous kind of death that signals the trauma of war and the indifference or failure of the institutions that are meant to care for the people who fight it. Of course, suicide is not just a matter of its representation—it is an irreducibly urgent problem in the lives of service members and their communities: In my ethnographic research over the past ten or so years with current and former service members and their families, care providers, and advocates, discussion of and experience with suicide are ubiquitous—self-inflicted death is now a central feature of how people experience contemporary war and tell their stories about it.

The topic of suicide is typically presented in terms of straightforward questions: What causes it and how can it be stopped? I argue that these questions can only be answered when they are placed in the context of the entire system of war-making that shapes soldiers' and veterans' experience. I describe that system here in terms of *military biopolitics*:

a set of institutional mechanisms and practices for disciplining soldiers' bodies and minds and empowering them to commit violence, and for deliberately exposing them to harm while also subjecting them to forms of control meant to keep them alive and effective as soldiers. The stresses that underlie military and veteran suicide are inextricably linked to this system of military biopolitics; so are efforts to surveil and prevent suicide and cultural attitudes about the meaning of service members' suffering, injury, and death. Military suicide presents the US public with a cultural problem: How are suicide deaths to be accounted for as simultaneously linked to war but also not the kind of "good death" we expect to be associated with it? American understandings of war death fixate on an imagined uniformed US fighter killed by the enemy in combat (Lutz 2013), but the proportion of deaths fitting that precise description—only a part of the approximately 7,000 or so US fatalities from the wars in Iraq and Afghanistan—are almost vanishingly small amidst a broader backdrop that also includes tens of thousands more contractor, coalition, and Iraqi and Afghan personnel, and hundreds of thousands of civilians. Attention to military suicide means attending to how war may affect its participants into the future, as service members struggle with mental illness and their families struggle to support them (or grieve their deaths), but, as another neglected category of war-related death, it also forces us to question who is included and excluded from our tallies of war's human costs.

Military Biopolitics and the Everyday Life of War-Making

Soldiers are subject to an extraordinary array of practices, rules, and institutional procedures that manage and organize their bodies and minds, heal, preserve, and care for them, make them disciplined tools of the state, empower them to kill, and deliberately expose them to harm. Borrowing from the philosopher Michel Foucault (2003), we can think of these practices, rules, and procedures as *military biopolitics*—a system of control governing how life and death are managed in military settings. This system defines the conditions under which, in Foucault's language, enemy lives are made to die or allowed to live, but also defines how American military are *allowed* to die and *made* to live (ibid.). The smooth functioning of military institutions depends on the discipline and reliability of soldiers' bodies and minds. Soldiers are in many ways defined by their capacity to complete physically and technically complex tasks, to master and respond reflexively to a complex regime of commands and orders, and to endure mental and physical pain without complaint or disruption. Many service members identify strongly and positively with these highly disciplined capacities that are intractably linked with the military's control over their minds and bodies (MacLeish 2013).

Some significant contradictions emerge here. The very activities that cultivate and prove soldiers' disciplined capacities—combat, war zone deployment, training, rigorous discipline, and the everyday labors of military life—also stress them out, exhaust them, and make them sick or injured. Medicine and diagnostic labels are thus a crucial aspect of military biopolitics' system of control. Military medicine, psychiatry, and public health, even as they serve the well-being of sick and injured soldiers, are also part of a system whose primary purpose is to keep a population of service members ready to engage in technically complex and physically demanding labor, exercise organized violence, and be exposed to harm. And if a soldier is too hurt or sick to do their job, it becomes a problem not just for them, but for the military institution as a whole. Suicide is just one extreme way that the organization's need for strong and compliant bodies and minds may be threatened by the limits, frailties, and vulnerabilities of human life. It is this reality that the US Army's 2010 suicide prevention report articulates in stating that the scale of military suicide has turned it from "a private affair or family matter" into a problem that "threatens our Army's readiness" (Department of the Army 2010).

A second contradiction arises from the fact that this biopolitics does not exist in a vacuum, but rather operates in conjunction with civilians' ambivalence about the injury and death that soldiers inflict and endure in their names. The military not only works to keep soldiers alive and healthy for its own purposes, but also to mollify the concerns of a civilian public with its own anxious investments in preventing service members' unnecessary suffering. Service members participate in violence in the name of (often bitterly contested) civilian political interests and in place of civilian bodies. Under the logic of military biopolitics, civilian guilt and complicity about harm befalling soldiers translates into an expectation that military institutions keep troops healthy and alive even as they are being exposed to harm. And it means that even as civilians take pride, satisfaction, or vicarious pleasure in troops' capacity to carry out violence, they may also worry about the military's ability to control that violence and ensure that it finds only appropriate outlets. Military suicide thus represents not only a real and urgent public health problem, but a double institutional failure—a perfect storm of cultural anxieties born of the logic of military biopolitics in which soldiers' lives are insufficiently cared for and their violence is insufficiently controlled.

Over the course of the wars in Iraq and Afghanistan, military and veteran suicide has become one of the primary signifiers of war-related stress and dysfunction, the subject of a full-blown moral panic rooted in these contradictions of military biopolitics (Wool 2014). But it is also an inescapable fact of life for those whose everyday labor makes war. In my conversations with soldiers, military families, care providers, and veterans, suicide is one of the first and most frequent points of reference for laying out the perceived stakes of war-related suffering, invoked with a frequency that would sound cliché were it not so incredibly grim. Everyone knows people who have killed themselves, often numerous people. Everyone who hasn't gone through it themselves knows many others who have struggled with despair, self-neglect, drug and alcohol use, and self-harm. I think of an acquaintance who almost never talks about her deployment without mentioning the story of a seemingly cheerful captain in her unit shooting himself in the head moments after he wished her good morning on their FOB in Afghanistan; or about a Marine vet and recovering meth addict who has had five guys from his old unit kill themselves; or about the young medic sexually assaulted by her commander who tried once with vodka and prescription sedatives and once by cutting her wrists, and survived both times; or about the outreach counselor and infantry vet who tells his clients to "stay busy if you don't wanna find yourself suck-starting a shotgun." The reality and the potential of self-inflicted death completely suffuse contemporary military and veteran life. As the next section of the chapter explains, the presumed link between combat-related trauma and suicide is not the only factor at work, and perhaps not even the main one. But as with other metrics of collective burden, like combat casualties or the military divorce rate, it was taken as given that all suicide was "war-related," because even for those who had come home and those who never deployed, war was the inescapable stuff of daily life. The frustrated declamation "And they wonder why soldiers are killing themselves!" would follow the denouement of a story about an extended deployment, a bad commander, a horrific injury, or a soldier's stressed-out family. The "they" in that statement is a reminder that this kind of death is defined by public scrutiny and attention. In holding up suicide as a routine occurrence, even when they are just talking to one another, folks in military communities are expressing a logical outcome of the grind of military biopolitics while also indicting the voyeuristic indifference of military and political leaders and the civilian public.

Rising Rates of Military Suicide

In modern times, suicide is literally defined by numbers. The invention of the suicide rate is a relatively recent phenomenon. It was born of state bureaucracies counting and statistically measuring citizens beginning in the mid-1800s, making self-inflicted death something that could be measured at the population level and objectifying it as a problem upon which government and medical experts could intervene (Hacking 2008; Marsh 2013). In the intervening 150 years, the suicide rate has come more or less to define contemporary understandings of suicide. The personal magnitude of a single individual suicide may be overwhelming for those affected by it, but it is the rise and fall of quantities and statistical indexes that are understood to reveal the urgency of suicide as a problem. These numbers offer aggregates and averages, but they say little about the subjective experience of suicidal people. And they are premised on the necessarily limited demographic factors it is possible to account for in a standardized forensic report, factors that may or may not take account of the complex structural contexts in which suicides occur. Military suicides may be "related to" war or military service, but what factors do leaders, policymakers, and the public look for to make sense of that relationship, and which ones do they potentially ignore?

It is clear from the available data that the number of self-inflicted deaths among active-duty military personnel has indeed risen steadily since 2003, reaching a high of 349 in 2012 (Department of the Army 2010, 2012) and then leveling off at between 250 and 300 deaths annually since then (see figure 9.1) (Associated Press 2013). As part of this trend, the suicide rate in the hardest-hit branches—the Army and the Marines—peaked at around twenty-three per 100,000 in 2012 (and again, declining slightly in the years since), surpassing an age- and gender-adjusted civilian rate of approximately eighteen per 100,000 (Department of the Army 2012). These figures do not include suicides in the Reserve and National Guard components, where rates have also climbed steadily and are sometimes dramatically higher than among active-duty troops (Hoge and Castro 2012),[2] nor do they include suicides among the approximately 2.5 million recent veterans of the wars in Iraq and Afghanistan. The bulk of military suicide deaths have occurred in the US Army—the largest of the service branches, and the one with the most substantial on-the-ground presence throughout the wars in Iraq and Afghanistan—but the Marines, also heavily taxed by on-the-ground demands, have experienced a high proportion as well, and suicides across all service branches are higher than they were in 2003 (Tan 2012a).[3]

Lengthy and repeated deployments—twelve to fifteen months long for the Army and often separated by less than a year in between—were a major and well-documented source of stress for service members (Howell and Wool 2011; Hautzinger and Scandlyn 2014; Tanielian and Jaycox 2008). Scholars and policymakers analyzing military suicide have generally assumed that it is driven by mental illnesses arising from or exacerbated by the strains of lengthy and repeated war-zone sojourns (Hoge and Castro 2012), including the acute fear and danger associated with combat conditions, the cumulative effects of everyday stress, and burdens on family and intimate relationships from long and repeated absences. Military leaders themselves acknowledge that the strain of prolonged and repeated deployments and a lack of behavioral health resources have "pushed some units, Soldiers and Families to the brink," in the words of one Army report (Hoge and Castro 2012, 1). The typical suicidal soldier, from this perspective, is a combat vet exhausted by multiple deployments and suffering from a diagnosable war-related mental illness.

However, military suicide data present some puzzling patterns. Studies based on data collected on service member suicides that occurred during military service showed that military suicides were most prevalent among service members who had deployed only once or not at all,

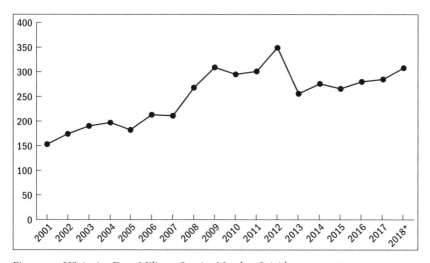

Figure 9.1. US Active Duty Military Service Member Suicides 2011–2018.
*Partial year
Source: Defense Casualty Analysis System, Department of Defense Suicide Event Reports, and Defense Suicide Prevention Office

and were especially elevated among those who left the military prematurely (Leard-Mann et al. 2013). The proportion of suicides among those with two or more deployments has risen and fallen in recent years, following no clear pattern (Associated Press 2013; Tan 2012b), but service members who never deployed at all account for almost a third of suicides from 2005 to 2010 (Gibbs and Thompson 2012). Analyses that include suicides after the conclusion of military service by combining multiple datasets present the counterintuitive finding that neither war-zone deployments (single or multiple) nor diagnosis with PTSD emerge statistically as risk factors for military suicide (Kang et al. 2015; Leard-Mann et al. 2013; Shen, Cunha, and Williams 2016). Various studies have found that the statistically "typical" military suicide is a junior enlisted white male in his early twenties who may have sought treatment or screened positively for symptoms of depression, anxiety, or substance abuse (Department of the Army 2010; National Center for Telehealth and Technology (T2), and Defense Centers of Excellence for Psychological Health and Traumatic Brain Injury (DCoE) 2012, 2013, 2014). The precipitating stressors include a combination of problems most often related to family and intimate relationships and financial and work-related difficulties (Department of the Army 2010; National Center for Telehealth and Technology 2014). In other words, from the perspective of the categories used to assess suicide at the population level, the typical military suicide looks a lot like the typical service member, but also, according to data from the Centers for Disease Control (Centers for Disease Control and Prevention 2012), a lot like the typical American civilian suicide.

Such findings have been presented by the media and by researchers themselves as indicating that there is "no link between combat deployment and suicides" (Kime 2015) or that "military-specific variables" are not responsible for the increase in incidence (Leard-Mann et al. 2013). But these assertions, while they provide an important challenge to commonsense assumptions about military suicide, are potentially misleading if we allow them to tell the entire story. First, as sociologist Stefan Timmermans writes, statistical claims like these "are far removed from either the smell of death or the memories of the living" (Timmermans 2007), boiling down lives that ended in self-inflicted death to an aggregate derived from a scant handful of demographic attributes, and often with little consideration for the multilevel interaction or broader systemic origins of those attributes (Krieger 1994; Wray, Colen, and Pescosolido 2011). The fact that deployment or military experiences do not reliably predict suicide in the aggregate does not mean that such things are unrelated to the actual military suicides that do occur—substantial portions of military suicides examined in recent studies occurred among service members who had deployed. Second, as anthropologist Emily Sogn points out, military data suggesting that non-war-related stressors like strained relationships or financial crises might be the most proximate impetus for suicides offer no basis on which to judge whether military life and aggressive operational tempo contribute to these issues (Sogn 2013). Recent scholarship on everyday military life suggests that stressful work and relationship problems born of the recent wars' relentless operation tempo typify contemporary military life rather than somehow lying outside the realm of "military-specific variables" (Finley 2011; MacLeish 2013; Wool 2015). Finally, the narrow focus on the links between suicide and deployment may miss the ways that the work of war and the elevated operational tempo of the wars in Iraq and Afghanistan strain the entire breadth of the military and reach far beyond the battlefield. A 2013 study found that rates of accidental injury and death among non-deployed personnel increased "in a way similar to suicide" over the mid-2000s (National Institute of Mental Health 2011a), highlighting the fact that making war is dangerous and stressful work even for those who do not deploy or experience combat.

One way to look at military suicide rates, then, is that they are not completely determined by the stresses of war individually or in the aggregate, but neither are they completely separable from those stresses. Instead of ruling out war-related factors as an explanation for suicide, the puzzling case of military suicide can lead us to rule *in* attention to the complexities of military biopolitics, a system in which the many different aspects of service members' lives—deployment, family, work—are deeply entangled rather than clearly separable.

Suicide Interventions

The Pentagon and the individual service branches have responded to the rise in suicides with a degree of initiative and transparency that belie any sense that they are trying to deny it or cover it up. Indeed, in recent years the military's own research and interventions have drawn as much attention to military suicide as have activists or the media. The military has gathered data to identify suicide risk factors that include mental illness diagnosis, drug and alcohol abuse, and criminality (Department of the Army 2010, 2012). It has issued public reports, mandated awareness trainings, and increased the availability of behavioral healthcare (Farmer 2013; Vogel 2012). All the while, it has, along with many political and media commentators, tried to eliminate stigma around help-seeking and to promote "culture change" to the institutional norms that prize individual endurance and fortitude above all else, sometimes to a fault (Miller and Bellon 2012; Tan 2012b).

The meaning and effectiveness of such efforts must be understood in the context of military biopolitics, in which a service member who suddenly cannot do their job or unexpectedly needs help immediately becomes a *problem* for their leaders, comrades, and care providers. It is not for nothing that troops sidelined by injury or illness are referred to (even by themselves) as "broken," no longer able to perform the standardized duties that define their role and usefulness (MacLeish 2013, 112). This is not just the result of individual callousness or even military cultural norms that scorn weakness, but rather a central feature of military life, especially under the aggressive operational tempo of wartime, and it is a pressure that troops feel keenly (103–116).

With suicide, this brokenness becomes intertwined with the notion of *risk*. As in public health more generally, military suicide prevention is framed in terms of monitoring "risky" behaviors, circumstances, and warning signs, including drug and alcohol abuse, criminality, and reckless behavior like fighting or driving too fast (Department of the Army 2010, 2012). When the urgency surrounding military suicide meets the logic of military biopolitics, however, such manifestations of troops' potential suffering may be treated by leaders and commanders as behavioral disruptions to be policed and managed rather than signs of more fundamental distress. Somewhat paradoxically, some of this literature, like the Army's 2010 and 2012 risk reduction reports, describes receipt of outpatient and inpatient behavioral health as part of an escalating set of "risky" attributes that culminate in criminality, violence, and suicide, even as these same documents emphasize the importance of help-seeking and reducing the stigma of diagnosis and treatment (Department of the Army 2010, 2012). Soldiers who have been "placed at risk" by the stresses of deployment become "risks" in themselves.

During my research at the Army's Fort Hood in 2007–08, I met soldiers who took seriously the prevalence of suicide among their fellows but grumbled about being reprimanded, placed under surveillance, and in one case even sent home from Iraq for making ill-advised exasperated remarks about harming themselves (MacLeish 2013, 227). Suicide "awareness" measures like this wallet-sized Army Public Health Service card (see figure 9.2) that were common sights at Fort Hood enlist soldiers to imagine one another—and themselves—as potentially "risky" subjects in need of intervention and control. Such injunctions leave soldiers at an impasse when military biopolitics demands their compliance and military cultural norms demand that they avoid seeking help or giving voice to their pain or worry.[4] Recent journalistic

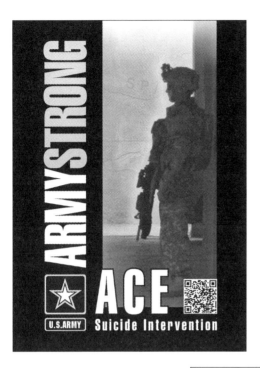

Figure 9.2. Suicide Prevention Wallet Card, Army Public Health Service

Ask your buddy
- Have the courage to ask the question, but stay calm
- Ask the question directly: Are you thinking of killing yourself?

Care for your buddy
- Calmly control the situation; do not use force; be safe
- Actively listen to show understanding and produce relief
- Remove any means that could be used for self-injury

Escort your buddy
- Never leave your buddy alone
- Escort to chain of command, Chaplain, behavioral health professional, or primary care provider
- Call the National Suicide Prevention Lifeline

National Suicide Prevention Lifeline:
1-800-273-8255(TALK) PRESS "1" for the Veteran's Crisis Line

USAPHC http://phc.amedd.army.mil/

TA - 095 - 0510

accounts suggest that even in the present risk-attentive climate, it is still possible for leaders to ignore signs of trouble or for service members actively seeking help to remain unable to get it before lethal despair overtakes them.[5]

At its best, the public alarm and official concern with military suicide, still a relatively rare phenomenon at the population level, could bring attention to the far more widespread stresses faced by the vast majority of service members. Military analyses and established suicidology findings do bear out the notion that suicide attempts and suicidal ideation are important risk factors to pay attention to, and intensive intervention like compulsory hospitalization can save service members' lives (Wool 2015). But as the military itself admits (Associated Press 2013; Tan 2012a, 2012b), the effectiveness of many education and awareness efforts remains unstudied and essentially unknown (Hoge and Castro 2012). And there are consequences to the tendency in public sentiment and military practice to gravitate to the worst-case scenario, dressed in a language of "crisis" and "epidemic" (Associated Press 2013; Briggs 2013; Morrison 2012) that suicide prevention advocates actually discourage (National Institute of Mental Health 2011b). Military mental health experts Charles Hoge and Carl Castro note that the absolutist rhetoric popular in military settings of "zero tolerance" for suicide or "just one" being "too many" stigmatizes the suicidal as individual failures or deviants and promotes a fantasy that all suicides can be prevented (Hoge and Castro 2012). Screening and prevention measures for high-risk conditions like suicide can also backfire when they are deployed outside of specialized mental health settings. This sense of elevated stakes can generate unnecessary referrals, reproduce stigma by linking common problems to the extremity and transgression of suicide, and undermine patients' trust in mental health care (ibid.). Hoge and Castro note that, while more investigation remains to be done, the most effective anti-suicide measures are means restriction (limiting easy access to tools of self-harm by, for instance, encouraging the use of trigger locks on guns or dispensing dangerous medications in small, single-dose portions), increased access to care (via rapid referral or hotlines), and psychosocial interventions like cognitive or dialectical behavioral therapy (Hoge and Castro 2012). Rather than simply looking to pathologized, individualized risk factors, these suggestions point to a systemic approach that demands reckoning with the everyday burdens of making war and the institutional environment within which service members live.

Stereotype, Suicide, and Public Perception

Focusing excessively on suicide may unintentionally set a high and narrow threshold for what is worthy of attention and intervention when it comes to the many complex burdens that confront military service members. This focus may allow the broader implications of military biopolitics to fade into the background or take on the status of unquestioned common sense. The cumulative stress of deployment, work demands, physical wear and tear, strain on family relationships, relocation, loss, and grief, among numerous other costs of war, are not given sufficient weight if they are reduced to mere warning signs for the ultimate threat of suicide. That is, this long list of problems persists even in the absence of suicide.

As I mentioned at the outset, the bigger stakes of this problem include not only the institutional arrangements in which service members' lives are embedded, but also the system of narratives and cultural assumptions that assign value and meaning to those lives. American representations of military service members frequently hew to an array of stereotypes that link the violence of war and military discipline to troops' presumed heroism and virtue, their exploitation and manipulation by the military, or their menacing deviance, pathology, and propensity for violence. In public culture, soldiers appear as sacrificing heroes deserving of special recognition, duped victims who have been deeply harmed by their service, or violent and mentally unstable threats to the peaceful social order they are meant to protect—stereotypes that mediate civilians' anxieties, fantasies, and ambivalence about the uncomfortably taboo and transgressive violence that service members commit in civilians' name (Kinder 2015; Lutz 2001; MacLeish 2009, 2013, 2014; Messinger 2008; Scandlyn and Hautzinger 2013; Wool 2015). Everything from the iconic traumas of Vietnam War films to media coverage of violent crimes or suicides committed by today's newest veterans contributes to the haze of pity, anxiety, and fear that swirls around images of service members.[6]

Public concerns about suicide epitomize these dynamics, stirring guilt, grief, and suspicion of the military and government (e.g., Kristof 2012) but also invoking the stereotypical figure of the "crazy vet"—a damaged, vulnerable victim capable of deadly violence toward others and themselves, a nightmarish inversion of the disciplined and carefully protected subject of military biopolitics (MacLeish 2009, 2014). Even as the stereotype pathologizes all soldiers, it focuses attention on a narrow set of extreme behaviors, actually making it harder to see the broader and subtler range of burdens that war inevitably places on those whose job it is to produce it. And when civilians wonder about how soldiers live with the unthinkable things we imagine them to have experienced, some fantasy of the suicidal soldier potentially offers a resolution, for it attests that ultimately they cannot live with those things (MacLeish 2013, 227). Suicide not only conceals the broader challenges confronting service members, but also provides an alibi that distances the public from their travails, reducing the latter to the exceptional or unfathomable deeds of combat rather than acknowledging the vast apparatus of routinized military violence in which the whole nation participates, often enthusiastically. As the editors of this volume point out in the conclusion, war rends the fabric of community. And yet, as so much of the work here also shows, "community" in the contemporary United States is inseparable from the waging of war (see Terry 2017): as a nation we are collectively comforted by warmaking, we perform our befuddled regret over it together, and we are bound by the ways we continue to fuel it.

It is for this reason that while the military and its ruthlessly instrumental treatment of human life may be the easiest villain to name in this story, it is disingenuous to let the buck stop there. For, just as service members are constrained by the military, the military is constrained as well: by the imperative to wage indefinite war with overwhelming force; by composing that force completely of volunteer soldiers; by abiding cultural notions that cover the soldier with unimpeachable glory and unexamined sentiment that may not translate well into real life; by worry over how the government can or should provide for its inevitably damaged servants (and whether it can afford to do so). But responsibility for these determining influences ultimately begins and ends with the people in whose name war is waged. Treatment and prevention programs are doubtless essential, as are changes to military culture. But most important of all may be changing our imagination of what war violence is and where it comes from. From this perspective, military suicide provides opportunities: to look sensitively and curiously at service members' experiences and the institutions that care for them rather than imagining them as pitiable, threatening, or already lost; and to think about war's effects on human survival and flourishing as arising not just from enemies and existential threats, but from systems that subject human life to harm routinely and on purpose.

NOTES

I am grateful to a number of funding sources for support of the research described here. Support came from a National Science Foundation Graduate Research Fellowship, a University of Texas University Fellowship, a Mental Health Services Research Traineeship from National Institute of Mental Health, a Vanderbilt University Research Scholar Faculty Development Grant, and a Wenner-Gren Foundation Post-PhD Research Grant.

1 Military suicide data are only available from the early 1980s onward. The low rate is attributable to the relative youth and good health of the military population, what epidemiologists call the "healthy worker" effect, as well as to the ready availability of healthcare and mental health resources (Hoge and Castro 2012, 671–672).

2 The frequency of suicide in the Reserve and National Guard components of the military—which in some branches, like the Army, are almost as large as the Active Duty component—has both fluctuated more over the long term and risen more in recent years (Kime 2016; Vazquez 2018). Guard and Reserve personnel may be especially vulnerable to post-deployment stress because they often return home to civilian communities devoid of specialized military mental health services and of military fellowship.

3 The Marine Corps, also especially heavily burdened by the wars, saw a 50 percent increase in suicides in 2011 (Tan 2012b) and a record 10-year high in 2018 (Snow 2019). Fewer Naval and Air Force personnel have deployed to Iraq and Afghanistan, and suicides in these services have not climbed as steadily or as dramatically. Statements from the military, Defense Department spokespersons, journalists, and commentators have characterized the suicide rate in different ways at different times, sometimes counting within individual service branches and other times across the whole military (Tan 2012b).

4 Erin Finley notes that this tension between being encouraged to seek help on the one hand and to "suck it up" on the other has been a central feature of military mental health care since the very beginning of the most recent wars (Finley 2011).

5 For example, Gibbs and Thompson's journalistic account tells the stories of an Army doctor who killed himself after his commander ignored entreaties from his wife that he needed help, and of an Apache helicopter pilot who committed suicide after unsuccessfully seeking counseling on multiple occasions (Gibbs and Thompson 2012; Wool 2015).

6 The shooting of former Navy SEAL sniper Chris Kyle by a fellow vet diagnosed with PTSD is only one prominent example (depicted in the 2014 movie, *American Sniper*). See, e.g., Alvarez 2008; Phillips 2009; Sontag and Alvarez 2008.

REFERENCES

Alvarez, L. 2008. "Army and Agency Will Study Rising Suicide Rate Among Soldiers." *New York Times*. October 30. Retrieved from www.nytimes.com.

Associated Press. 2013. "2012 Military Suicides Hit Record High of 349." January 14. Retrieved from bigstory.ap.org.

Briggs, B. 2013. "Military Suicide Rate Hit Record High in 2012." January 14. Retrieved from usnews.nbcnews.com.

Centers for Disease Control and Prevention. 2012. "At a Glance—Statistics—Suicide." May 11. Retrieved from www.cdc.gov.

Department of the Army. 2010. *Army Health Promotion/Risk Reduction/Suicide Prevention Report 2010*. Washington, DC: US Department of the Army. Retrieved from usarmy.vo.llnwd.net.

Department of the Army. 2012. *Army 2020: Generating Health and Discipline in the Force Ahead of the Strategic Reset*. Washington, DC: US Department of the Army. Retrieved from usarmy.vo.llnwd.net.

Farmer, B. 2013. "To Combat Suicides, Army Focuses on the Homefront." *All Things Considered*. Retrieved from www.npr.org.

Finley, E. P. 2011. *Fields of Combat: Understanding PTSD Among Veterans of Iraq and Afghanistan*. Ithaca, NY: Cornell University Press.

Foucault, M. 2003. *Society Must Be Defended: Lectures at the Collège de France, 1975–76*, edited by M. Bertani and A. Fontana; translated by D. Macey. New York: Picador.

Gibbs, N., and M. Thompson. 2012. "The War on Suicide?" *Time*, July 23. Retrieved from www.time.com.

Hacking, I. 2008. "The Suicide Weapon." *Critical Inquiry* 35(1): 1–32. doi.org/10.1086/595626.

Hautzinger, S., and J. Scandlyn. 2014. *Beyond Posttraumatic Stress: Homefront Struggles with the Wars on Terror*. Walnut Creek, CA: Left Coast Press.

Hoge, C., and C. Castro. 2012. "Preventing Suicides in US Service Members and Veterans: Concerns After a Decade of War." *JAMA* 308(7): 671–672. doi.org/10.1001/jama.2012.9955.

Howell, A., and Z. H. Wool. 2011. "The War Comes Home: The Toll of War and the Shifting Burden of Care." Retrieved from http://watson.brown.edu/costsofwar.

Kang, H. K., T. A. Bullman, D. Smolenski, N. A. Skopp, G. A. Gahm, and M. A. Reger. 2015. "Suicide Risk among 1.3 Million Veterans Who Were on Active Duty during the Iraq and Afghanistan Wars." *Annals of Epidemiology* 25(2): 96–100. doi.org/10.1016/j.annepidem.2014.11.020.

Kime, P. 2015. "Study: No Link between Combat Deployment and Suicides." *Military Times*, April 1. Retrieved from www.militarytimes.com.

Kime, Patricia. 2016. "Reserve Suicides Up 23 Percent—Active-Duty Count Remains Steady." *Military Times*, April 4. Retrieved from www.militarytimes.com.

Kinder, J. M. 2015. *Paying with Their Bodies: American War and the Problem of the Disabled Veteran*. Chicago: University of Chicago Press.

Krieger, N. 1994. "Epidemiology and the Web of Causation: Has Anyone Seen the Spider?" *Social Science and Medicine* 39(7): 887–903. doi.org/10.1016/0277-9536 (94)90202-X.

Kristof, N. D. 2012. "A Veteran's Death, the Nation's Shame." *New York Times*, April 14. Retrieved from www.nytimes.com.

Leard-Mann, C. A., T. M. Powell, T. C. Smith, M. R. Bell, B. Smith, E. J. Boyko, . . . C. W. Hoge. 2013. "Risk Factors Associated with Suicide in Current and Former US Military Personnel." *JAMA* 310(5): 496. doi.org/10.1001/jama.2013.65164.

Lutz, C. 2001. *Homefront: A Military City and the American Twentieth Century*. Boston: Beacon Press.

Lutz, C. 2013. "US and Coalition Casualties in Iraq and Afghanistan." Retrieved from http://watson.brown.edu/costsofwar.

MacLeish, K. 2009. "Wounds of War and the Dilemmas of Stereotype." *Savage Minds*, September 27. Retrieved from savageminds.org.

MacLeish, K. 2013. *Making War at Fort Hood: Life and Uncertainty in a Military Community*. Princeton, NJ: Princeton University Press.

MacLeish, K. 2014. "The Ethnography of Good Machines." *Critical Military Studies* 1(1): 11–22. doi.org/10.1080/23337486.2014.973680.

Marsh, I. 2013. "The Uses of History in the Unmaking of Modern Suicide." *Journal of Social History* 46(3): 744–756.

Messinger, S. 2008. "What Do We Owe Them: Veterans, Disability and the Privatization of American Civic Life." *Journal of Religion, Disability and Health* 12(3): 267–286. doi.org/10.1080/15228960802269398.

Miller, C., and P. Bellon. 2012. "The U.S. Army Can't Stop Soldiers from Killing Themselves." *Atlantic*, October 12. Retrieved from www.theatlantic.com.

Morrison, M. 2012. "Suicide Crisis: Why the Military Needs Mandatory Mental-Health Services." *Daily Beast*, September 27. Retrieved from www.thedailybeast.com.

National Center for Telehealth and Technology (T2), and Defense Centers of Excellence for Psychological Health and Traumatic Brain Injury (DCoE). 2012. *Department of Defense Suicide Event Report—Calendar Year 2011 Annual Report*. Washington, DC: T2 and DCoE. Retrieved from www.t2.health.mil.

National Center for Telehealth and Technology (T2), and Defense Center of Excellence for Psychological Health and Traumatic Brain Injury (DCoE). 2013. *Department of Defense Suicide Event Report—Calendar Year 2012 Annual Report*. Washington, DC: T2 and DCoE. Retrieved from www.t2.health.mil.

National Center for Telehealth and Technology (T2), and Defense Centers of Excellence for Psychological Health and Traumatic Brain Injury (DCoE). 2014. *Department of Defense Suicide Event Report—Calendar Year 2013 Annual Report*. Washington, DC: T2 and DCoE. Retrieved from www.t2.health.mil.

National Institute of Mental Health. 2011a. NIMH Army STARRS Preliminary Data Reveal Some Potential Predictive Factors for Suicide. Retrieved from www.nimh.nih.gov.

National Institute of Mental Health. 2011b. Recommendations for Reporting on Suicide. Retrieved from www.nimh.nih.gov.

Phillips, D. 2009. "Casualties of War, Part I: The Hell of War Comes Home." *Colorado Springs Gazette*, July 25. Retrieved from www.gazette.com.

Scandlyn, J., and S. Hautzinger. 2013. "Collective Reckoning with the Post-9/11 Wars on a Colorado Homefront." Retrieved from http://watson.brown.edu/costsofwar.

Shen, Y.-C., J. M. Cunha, and T. V. Williams. 2016. "Time-varying Associations of Suicide with Deployments, Mental Health Conditions, and Stressful Life Events among Current and Former US Military Personnel: A Retrospective Multivariate Analysis." *The Lancet Psychiatry* 3(11): 1039–1048. https://doi.org.

Snow, S. 2019. "The Corps' Suicide Rate Is At a 10-year High. This Is How the Marines Plan to Address It." *Marine Corps Times*. Retrieved from marinecorpstimes.com.

Sogn, E. 2013. "War Death and Epidemiological Imagination." *Somatosphere*, December 4. Retrieved from www.somatosphere.net.

Sontag, D., and L. Alvarez. 2008. "War Torn: Coverage by Deborah Sontag and Lizette Alvarez." *New York Times*. Retrieved from topics.nytimes.com.

Tan, M. 2012a. "Overall Suicides Down 10 Percent for 2011." *Army Times*, January 30. Retrieved from www.armytimes.com.

Tan, M. 2012b. "In Suicides, Army Faces Steepest Challenge." *Army Times*, September 25. Retrieved from www.armytimes.com.

Tanielian, T., and L. Jaycox. 2008. *Invisible Wounds of War: Psychological and Cognitive Injuries, Their Consequences, and Services to Assist Recovery*. Santa Monica, CA: RAND Corporation.

Terry, J. 2017. *Attachments to War: Biomedical Logics and Violence in Twenty-First-Century America*. Durham, NC: Duke University Press.

Timmermans, S. 2007. *Postmortem: How Medical Examiners Explain Suspicious Deaths*. Chicago: University of Chicago Press.

Vazquez, Rennie. 2018. "Department of Defense (DoD) Quarterly Suicide Report (QSR) 1st Quarter, CY 2018." Washington, DC: Defense Suicide Prevention Office. Retrieved from http://www.dspo.mil.

Vogel, S. 2012. "Army Stands Down Thursday to Focus on Suicide Prevention." *Washington Post*, September 26. Retrieved from www.washingtonpost.com.

Wool, Z. 2014. "Critical Military Studies, Queer Theory, and the Possibilities of Critique: The Case of Suicide and Family Caregiving in the US Military." *Critical Military Studies* 1(1): 23–37. doi.org/10.1080/23337486.2014.964600.

Wool, Z. 2015. *After War: The Weight of Life at Walter Reed*. Durham, NC: Duke University Press.

Wray, M., C. Colen, and B. Pescosolido. 2011. "The Sociology of Suicide." *Annual Review of Sociology* 37(1): 505–528. doi.org/10.1146/annurev-soc-081309-150058.

10

Afterwar Work for Life

ZOË H. WOOL

Though the exact numbers are hard to come by, as of this writing roughly 1 million post–9/11 veterans need or have sought care for a service-connected injury or illness.[1] Talk of injured veterans tends to conjure that most iconic image of the war-injured soldier: a young man missing a limb but otherwise unscathed by his time in combat. But such images can be deceiving (and not only because women constitute an increasing proportion of veterans). Take, for example, the details of injury. Amputations themselves are far from simple injuries, requiring a lifetime of maintenance, adjustment, and care. They are not "over" if a veteran walks away from a hospital on a prosthetic leg. And they rarely occur in isolation: In these wars where 60 percent of injuries are caused by Improvised Explosive Devices (IEDs), amputations are usually only the most dramatic of an array of injuries resulting from a single injuring event, including burns, broken bones, shrapnel wounds, ruptured eardrums, concussion, and traumatic brain injury (TBI). What's more, while that image of the war veteran amputee and the simplified picture of his injury may be the most iconic, amputations account for only a tiny fraction of war injuries in the current era: All told, the post–9/11 wars in Iraq and Afghanistan have led to fewer than 2,000 amputations among US service members. So what, then, is a more accurate picture? What are the ailments for which veterans are seeking care? And if that care does not conform to the cultural and biomedical fantasy of the clean cure of prosthetic technology (Terry 2017), what does it look like? The answers offer, in some ways, a much more banal picture.

Alejandro, a veteran in his late thirties, has an 80 percent disability rating for a combination of PTSD, asthma, depression, and a slew of low-grade chronic orthopedic issues. He is married, and a father of two sons, one of whom was born while he was deployed. He can no longer work, and struggles with binge drinking, which has exacerbated his health conditions, including diabetes. Jane is a veteran in her early forties who has a 70 percent disability rating for chronic stomach and eye problems, broken ankles, depression, and sometimes debilitating back pain. She is a single mother of one, and works part time as an occupational therapist. Ryan is in his mid-thirties and has a 30 percent disability rating for tinnitus, PTSD, and back pain and is trying to get his knee pain and sinus problems included in his rating. He uses a CPAP machine to help him breathe when he sleeps, and though he expected he might eventually need one given his family history, he is certain that his military service is responsible for effectively accelerating the aging of his body by what seems decades. Among the most common ailments suffered by veterans is chronic joint and back pain, sometimes associated with combat-related events like those caused by IEDs, but often (and sometimes also) associated with the considerable daily wear and tear that the body takes when it is required to carry an extra 60–100 pounds of armor for weeks and months at a time (see MacLeish 2013). The next most common are those struggles with daily life that register as diagnoses of mental illness. PTSD is most common among them and has been diagnosed in about 20 percent of veterans, followed closely by depression and anxiety.[2] Since 2001, 36,850 veterans have been diagnosed with TBI.[3] Often, veterans struggling with one of these issues are also struggling with others, and so, like Alejandro, Jane, and Ryan, they frequently end up with multiple diagnoses for chronic conditions.

This preponderance of multiple diagnoses is hardly surprising, a function of both the complexity of war-related debility and the technology of diagnosis itself. Clinical encounters sort what is experienced as the unruly mess of life and pain into discrete diagnostic categories, lumping together nightmares and anger, separating out sleeplessness, distinguishing these from aching vertebrae. While often helpful, these diagnostic schema are never quite up to the task of capturing the complexity of life as it is lived (Wool 2013). To be sure, by naming these experiences, diagnoses help organize them and chart a course for clinical treatment. But just as the complexity of life exceeds diagnostic categories, so does much of the living with these conditions extend beyond the space of the clinic: A medication may be prescribed in the clinic, but it must be taken and managed at home. A regime of talk or behavioral therapy may offer a space or technique to productively engage with debilitating or dysfunctional emotions, behaviors, or relationships, but it may be beyond your grasp when you are seized by panic while driving in your car. One veteran I knew, Alex, had received a disability rating from the VA entitling him to treatment for the damage to his spine which he sustained as a result of the routines of relatively uneventful army service spent mostly on a Forward Operating Base in the early years of the Iraq war. But his diagnosis and medical care were of little help as he attempted to navigate his life with chronic and worsening pain, unsure if he would be able to get out of bed from one day to the next and certain that he would be unable to walk by the time he reached age forty. More than the iconic injuries that are publicly glorified as they are transformed into sanitized signs of sacrifice (Wool 2015, 109–13), this is how many veterans with war-torn bodies experience daily life.

It is in the nature of biomedical treatment that experiences of distress exceed it.[4] The forms of care it offers rely on a circumscribed and situated perspective that attends—often quite well—to certain forms of suffering, discomfort, and struggle that are legible at a specific, clinically relevant scale: the cell, the organ system, the body, or the individual. But, in the case of US veterans, as for so many others, this necessarily partial nature of clinical care is exacerbated by problems of institutional scarcity, when the need for particular forms of care exceeds the capacity or the capability or the mandate of the institution, in this case the VA. The 2014 VA scandal, touched off by allegations that dozens of veterans died while on waitlists to see doctors at the VA in Phoenix, Arizona, offers the most recent spectacularized example. Practices of delaying access or keeping names off of waitlists to make the lists seem shorter and give the appearance that the VA was able to keep up with veterans' needs led to a criminal investigation by the FBI as well as a separate White House investigation and the eventual resignation of then VA chairman General Shinseki (Oppel Jr. and Shear 2014). We might also recall the 2008 memo from the PTSD program coordinator at the Temple, Texas VA suggesting that clinicians should avoid diagnosing veterans with PTSD because it is costly and time-consuming and providing services to veterans diagnosed with PTSD was overtaxing institutional resources.[5] Beyond and beneath these headlines are the daily experiences of a subset of veterans I have encountered in recent years, those deemed "the most needy" by support organizations. These are veterans who, sometimes a decade after the end of their service in Iraq or Afghanistan, continue to struggle daily with pain, anxiety, depression, and not infrequently suicidality. For them, the VA is a source of aid. However, it is also a source of tremendous frustration both because of its notorious bureaucracy, which is laborious and depersonalizing to navigate, and because it often seems like a site of ceaseless investments in an elusive cure rather than facilitating the quieter, less aspirational, but sometimes more healthy arts of care.[6] Veterans may require daily care for decades and still feel powerfully compelled along the therapeutic odyssey toward the utopia of cure. Others may work to accommodate their new conditions but still seek out biomedical treatment and diagnostic answers in the search for the best quality of life. After years of bouncing from specialist to specialist and investigating every possible explanation for his illnesses, Devin received diagnoses of chronic fatigue syndrome, irritable bowel syndrome, fibromyalgia, and PTSD. He then made a rule that he and his husband Stephen would only pursue one new diagnosis or one new treatment at a time, because the crush of appointments, sorting out of paperwork, and juggling of medications was itself too draining. Many, like Devin, are unable to manage all of this on their own. And even those who do must contend with the pervasive social fantasy of the good life that insinuates a life worth living is one stabilized by the normative entailments of true love (Foucault 1990; Povinelli 2006). Bud, a veteran with severe PTSD and moderate TBI, had made a home for himself and his young son, who also had a degenerative muscular condition. He felt the thing he needed most of all was a wife. Without that, he wasn't sure how he'd be able to go on. Jason, a veteran with a severe penetrating TBI said getting a girlfriend was his number one therapeutic goal. Despite being generally quite happy with his life and his mother's excellent management of his care in the home that they share, he hinges his desired future to a wife and kids. In most ideals of liberalism, this fantasy of true love is seen as the best and most natural, even the most human (Kleinman 2010), relation of support for someone who is injured or ill. This fantasy is amplified in the military context, where normative visions of the family hold sway both during service and after (Wool 2016), and where, at the level of the institution, support for veterans' futures often comes packaged as support for the supposedly stabilizing form of a normative family life, the normative nuclear family.

When we reach the limits of institutional capacity, we encounter a familiar dynamic of biomedicine and attendant political economies of care and responsibility: When the institution cannot or does not provide the forms of care and support it deems necessary, responsibility for care is shifted elsewhere, sometimes to the individual, but very often (and sometimes also) to the family.[7] Sometimes this happens formally, through policies that stipulate family responsibility, and sometimes it happens informally, through powerful and socially supported moral expectations that family *should* be the space of care, and often a combination of the two. Among the current generation of injured veterans whose needs are so often chronic and diffused throughout their daily lives—whose bodies ache, whose heads throb, whose nights are tortured by fear—family is increasingly being transformed into the space of care and expected to function as a kind of annex to medical and military institutions, thrusting family members into the "grey zone of care where the labors of love mix with the work of medically managing life" (Wool and Messinger 2012, 44).

There are two essential points I would like to make about this situation. One is about the nature and force of the particular idea of family being turned into the space of care; and the second is about the nature and force of the particular idea of life being turned into the object of care.

Family

The archetype of *family* imagined in this care scheme is a very specific one, a normative configuration of a male injured veteran and his caregiving wife. The repeal of Don't Ask Don't Tell hasn't changed this scheme much, other than perhaps to make homonormative families more explicitly included, showing the nuclear family norm to be profoundly resilient and making it all the more clear that those outside its charmed circle are all the less sanctioned. The fact that an increasing number of male veterans' wives are themselves veterans escapes this imagination; as does the increasing number of female veterans; as does the abundance of single soldiers. In the ideal archetypical family form within which care is supposed to be sequestered, there may also be children, but the family is imagined as living all together by themselves, that is, a single nuclear family in a single-generation household. And at the core of this configuration is that familiar pair of most significant others: the conjugal couple (Povinelli 2006).[8] Injured veterans who don't fit this profile are subjected to it in various ways.

Devin and Steven, who married in 2013 and are planning to adopt a child, fit the profile quite well and almost never felt their providers made an issue of their gayness.[9] But Jane, who is petite, blond, preppy, and always neatly put together, had her veteran status challenged by a parking valet when she arrived at the VA's emergency entrance in the midst of an attack of acute pain, despite her disabled veteran license plates. Inside VA hospitals, she is also regularly mistaken for a caregiver by staff and other patients alike and is often sexualized and hit on by older male veterans. In dual veteran couples, when one person is a caregiver, their own veteran status is often eclipsed by their caregiver role, all the more so when the caregiving veteran is also a wife. During a retreat for injured veterans and caregivers, I was surprised to learn that Sharon, a caregiver who had been vocally sharing her experiences and frustrations with the group, was also a veteran. She hadn't mentioned her status at all during the first three days of the retreat, and she mentioned her veteran status to me only incidentally as she noted that her status gave her access to health insurance coverage for a variety of somaticizing symptoms of caregiving-related stress.

When families don't conform to the nuclear model, the results can be unpredictable. One Mexican American soldier at Walter Reed Army Medical Center had his mother, father, brother, and occasionally sister at his side while he went through years of rehabilitation, even though the Nonmedical Attendant program that supported the presence of family members as caregivers at Walter Reed only supported one family member per veteran at a time. Some saw this comparative abundance of family as a sign of commitment and support, though one that was problematically racialized, evidence of a stereotype of Mexican family values. Others, drawing on the same stereotype, saw it as evidence of an irrational and almost pathological multiplicity of relations and tied it to laziness and a culture of freeloading. In this way, the ideal family form is not only hetero- and homonormative, but also raced and classed in its attunement to a social and cultural norm of white middle-class domesticity.

There are few models of care that present alternatives to the family, posed, as it often is, as the only alternative to institutionalization and abandonment (Biehl 2005). Perhaps the most significant is the model of companionate and collective care, including hospice volunteerism, which developed in response to massive AIDS deaths in gay communities during the first decade of the AIDS crisis (Russ 2005). But while this model extends care beyond the family, it is primarily a model of care at the end of life rather than the long-term and generally consistent, rather than increasing, support many injured veterans require.

A model that may offer more relevant lessons is that of the disability care collective. The care collective is an umbrella term for an array of practices through which a self-organized network—often conceived of as chosen kin—participate in facilitating the daily needs of one or more people who need help, and in so doing, they also constitute something of a community or collective (McArthur 2014). Care collectives may be more or less formally organized; they may or may not involve self-organized communal living or barter; and their members may come and go with varying frequency. The most salient dimensions of these approaches to daily care are that they push back against the dyad of a single caregiver and care-receiver upon which most models of care—within the family or otherwise—are based (e.g., Kittay 1999). These models also situate needs within a broader context of collective social obligation, as opposed to models of caregiving that separate clinical needs from the relationships that help meet them, and prioritize the clinical over the relational or social. In these ways, care collectives are the opposite of the normative image of care for veterans, contained within the conjugal couple. Still other models can be found in Black feminist thought, which offers collectivity "as an alternative to the heteronormative domesticity that is the primary organizing social logic of the state" (Colbert 2013). Here, the collectivizing of care is a political maneuver that pushes back against the perverse racial logics of the Moynihan Report and its progeny, finding ways to recognize and regard the intimate socialities of

"African American families [that] historically assume configurations for which the dominant order has no category" (Cheryl Wade cited in Colbert 2013).[10]

The consequences of a public imaginary that sees non-clinical care for veterans as properly sequestered within a narrowly defined family are manifold. One is that the very relationships of love that are supposed to sustain care become strained by its burden, sometimes to the point of breaking. Another is that the moral imperative to care, and, more specifically, to care for the very lives of veterans, as I discuss below, can act as a compelling force, making it exceedingly difficult for people to uncouple their lives from each other, even when all other attachments have gone or when the ones that remain are violent or hazardous (Wool 2015, 182–86), or to relinquish or move on from this particular project of care or this iteration of family. Another is that the horizon of possibility for life, the array of social forms and modes of attention and practice and intimacy that secure, sustain, or buoy it, becomes narrowed. Certainly, there are many couples who, sometimes in spite of these pressures rather than because of them, make good lives while keeping care more or less contained. Devin and Stephen, for example, have moved through periods of confusion, despair, and resentment, and found themselves deeply devoted to each other and ready to become parents. Ana and David García had been married for many years before David became ill from exposure to toxic smoke from the massive open-air military waste burn pits he encountered during his deployment to Iraq.[11] As David's health deteriorated, and he was forced out of his civilian job as a highway patrolman, Ana threw herself into caring for him, and advocating for other ill and injured veterans. They continue to support each other in their ongoing struggle. But many others do not. A recent NPR story offered harrowing accounts of three women who were abused by their disabled veteran husbands while acting as their full-time caregivers, a care arrangement supported by VA programs for family caregiving (Lawrence 2016). Far more representative than the abuse in these cases is the way these women feel stuck in this arrangement of care, both because the VA caregiver support program pays them to stay, and because of the morally weighted social pressure to "support the troops" which, in these cases, means keeping care sequestered within a relationship that may be bad for everyone involved. Post–9/11 veterans' wives are especially compelled to take on and stay in the role of caregiver through policy initiatives and social expectation alike. They are also more likely than other caregivers to suffer from their own mental health problems and to have fewer social supports than their pre–9/11 veteran or civilian caregiver counterparts (Ramchand et al. 2014).

Despite the many consequences of the family care model for veterans, it is hardly surprising that this work of managing the extensive violence of war should leverage obligations of love and kin. After all, since the end of the draft in 1973, the military has ever more explicitly brought family into the ambit of war work as part of a concerted strategy to recruit and retain soldiers; an effort that involves both making the military family-friendly and making the family military-friendly. Military families are now considered part of the "Total Force" (Chu, Hall, and Jones 2007) and recognized as essential to the functioning and readiness of the military itself (Scandlyn and Hautzinger, in this volume). And the same is true for life after war. Clinical and political efforts to intervene in the scenes of afterwar suffering and distress now lean on family members of soldiers and veterans—particularly wives—in a way that is much more explicit and institutionalized than has historically been the case.

In the landscape of American military life that animates our post–9/11 wars, the work of maintaining the life of injured soldiers in the afterwar is routed through intimate attachments, particularly conjugal couplehood, like never before. The previous era's primary concern with transforming injured soldiers into wage-earning men has gradually been eclipsed by concerns to transform them into normatively sexually capacitated ones, with an increasing, and increasingly public, concern for their sexual anatomy and functioning (Wood 2012; Wool 2016), as well as for the heteronormative (or homonormative) social forms that are supposed to both contain and secure them. There are myriad factors that contribute to this historical shift, including: the disappearance of the family wage, requiring two wage earners to sustain a household; the general shifting cultural entailments of hegemonic masculinities away from the affectively cool (if sometimes violent) protectors and providers of twentieth-century patriarchy and toward more culturally and affectively enmeshed and anxious figures, more neoliberal consumers than Fordist producers, and more in the family than lording over it (see Connell 2005; Kimmel 2006; Watson and Shaw 2011); the end of the draft; the shrinking of the standing army; and the national reaction-formation to the public shaming of Vietnam veterans that has elevated and sacrilized combat-injured soldier bodies above even other soldier bodies, particularly in the post–9/11 era.

Each of these factors must itself be understood within broader material, social, and political fields, which always include articulations of a subject who is self-determining and self-responsible, as well as public structures of intimacy, that is, those socially conventionalized ideas about sexuality, gender, and intimate relations that frequently are the subject of public debate or control. Though a full elaboration is beyond the scope of this chapter, I highlight these factors because their convergence has shaped a social, cultural, and political space of afterwar life in the contemporary United States in which the valorized aspect of the veteran figure is ascendant (though still shadowed by the vilified one) (see Lutz 2001); public attention to and concern for the lives of injured veterans is especially valued; and the embrace of the injured veteran body within the loving arms of a caring spouse, when accompanied by the cultural trappings of the consumer class racially coded as white, can itself appear as a solution to the problem of injured soldier bodies. It can appear so especially in relation to the "dilemma of disabled masculinity" (Shuttleworth, Wedgwood, and Wilson 2012) that war produces.

For all these reasons, as the provisioning of care for veterans is being structured into "the family," it is the relation of husband and wife, or, less ideally, boyfriend and girlfriend, that is expected to bear the weight of care.

Life

In the current situation, it is a more or less biological, and almost exclusively bodily, life of the soldier that these ideally imagined wives and girlfriends are being called to attend to. This is a life whose vitality must be monitored and managed, with the task of caregiving taking on its more medicalized valiance. As experience is disaggregated into diagnostic categories, so the need for care, and care itself, is becoming attached to biomedical diagnoses. *Care* comes to name the practices through which symptoms, understood as such, are addressed. For example, the

VA Caregiver Support website now offers Diagnosis Care Sheets. "We know what you are thinking," the website reassures the anticipated caregiver reader:

> You don't speak Latin, and you don't have a medical degree. But you still need to understand the medical condition of the Veteran you care for and how to manage it. VA created plain-language care sheets to give you the bottom line on managing the medical condition for the Veteran you love.

At the same time, care maintains its less clinical and more intimate implications. After all, it is this sense of care, care as the obligation to another's body compelled by love rather than medical need, that ironically makes the family, and specifically the conjugal couple, appear so well suited to that other, more medicalized kind of care that the body requires. Love is precisely what is supposed to make *loved ones* good and proper caregivers. Perhaps, then, it is not surprising that alongside the Diagnosis Care Sheets for PTSD, TBI, and less war-bound conditions like ALS and Alzheimer's, there is *A Caregivers Guide to Intimacy*, with information on how war injury and homecoming can affect sex and physical intimacy, and how that intimate bodily problem of sex after war should be managed. In these ways, it is specifically the veteran's body that becomes the object of care, both as the site of clinical symptoms requiring care-as-symptom-management, and as the site of love requiring care-as-intimate-touch (Wool 2015).

One of the things that makes this situation of veterans distinctive from many others in which family members may be expected to care for injured, ailing, or otherwise debilitated loved ones is the way this dual focus on the body as the object of love and the subject of debility comes to a particularly sharp point against a backdrop of suicide that haunts the veteran of these recent wars: Through this perceived risk, the norm of conjugal care can come to be figured as the very difference between life and death.

A bit of background will help explain the relevance of suicide. While suicide rates among soldiers have consistently been lower than for their age- and gender-adjusted civilian counterparts (a point of pride for the military), soldier rates surpassed civilian rates in 2008 and remained historically high. In recent years, the problem of veteran suicide has also begun receiving broad attention and concern, with a recent VA report noting that over the last twelve years, rates of suicide among veterans of all eras have been relatively stable, at 18–20 per day. Most veterans who commit suicide are not veterans of post–9/11 wars, and not all those who commit suicide have service-connected diagnoses. Nonetheless, this widespread concern about military suicide has led to a "moral panic" (MacLeish 2012), and suicide has become ubiquitous as both a fear and expectation in efforts to address the needs of post–9/11 veterans who are struggling with afterwar life (MacLeish 2018; this volume). This shadow of concern for veterans' lives constantly understood as lives-at-risk hovers over the situation of conjugal care.

Afterwar Work for Life

As soldier and veteran suicides have become a matter of concern in an intractable way, major efforts are being made both to definitively understand why soldiers are killing themselves (a doomed task, as suicide researchers might themselves have sadly warned), and to prevent them from doing so. And in these attempts to salvage life from the grips of death, the archetype of the conjugal couple once again appears as a prime relation of care for life. Take the following example.

"The only reason he is alive," says Mike Yurchison, "is his girlfriend, Leigh Anna Landsberger." So begins a recent Nicholas Kristof column in the *New York Times*. "She gave Mike, 34, something to live for after his brother, an Iraq veteran confronting similar torment, died of a drug overdose, an apparent suicide. She talked him through his grief after the suicide of another Army buddy." Kristoff tells us. And what, we might ask, does she do to keep Mike alive now? "She sits with him through endless waits at the Veterans Affairs, whispering that he's smarter than she is even if his brain is damaged. She helps him through his seizures, and she nags him to overcome his drug addiction" (Kristof 2014).

This story represents an increasingly ubiquitous genre in the United States used in understanding life made precarious by the many forms of violence inherent to war and military life. This genre presents such intimacies within a morally persuasive framework of care and caregiving contained within the intimate embrace of couplehood. Most iterations, like this one, are starkly anti-political, presenting family caregiving as a moral good while bracketing the questions of why such caregiving is needed and if or why wives and girlfriends should be expected to do it.

This genre is not limited to humanistic narratives such as the one presented above. In fact, the bonds of couplehood appear across many attempts to quantitatively pinpoint the trajectories that lead to soldier suicide. For example, in statistical attempts to understand the causes of soldier and veteran suicide, "Relationship problems" appear as a consistent but vague mechanism bridging the diffuse strains of military life and the specified problem of military suicide. And a recent study looking at suicide in the National Guard found "a loss of significant other was related to increased suicide intentions after deployment" (Griffith and Vaitkus 2013, 643).[12]

Such disturbances were also framed as bound to suicide across the army's two major suicide reports, published in 2010 and 2012 (Chiarelli 2010, 2012). The reports include vignettes of suicidal cases in which divorce, domestic acrimony, or the lack of such relationships are prevalent features. And throughout the reports, there is an emphasis on family as an essential dimension of army life and an essential element in the management of suicide, for example, enumerating the "unit strand," the "soldier strand," and the "family strand" as the three inextricable elements of the "composite life cycle model" for understanding risky periods of life stress that increase risk of suicide. The much-touted Comprehensive Soldier Fitness program, rolled out across the army in 2009, largely in response to the joint problems of PTSD and suicide, is now officially called the Comprehensive Soldier and *Family* Fitness (CSF2).

What emerges across these very different attempts to understand and respond to soldier and veteran suicide is that if "loss of significant other" can put a veteran at risk for suicide, the presence of a significant other can shore up life. The others represented as most significant are nearly always girlfriends and wives. In the context of injury, the presence of such specific others itself shored up when they are expected to be present and accountable in the name of care.

In this context we might think of "care" as *afterwar work for life*. I mean afterwar *work for life* here both in the sense that the specter of suicide puts the very life of the body itself at stake in the labor and complex attachment that is glossed as "caregiving" and in the sense that "care" here is a form of intervention that is not curative but preventative and so is, by default, expected to last a long lifetime.[13]

The public expectation is that such work for life is and should be confined within the bonds of family. Spouses especially are "supported" into such work, both through the force of normative expectations and through programs like the VA caregiver support program which was created in 2010 to support this work on the assumption that those doing it would be spouses. The program offers concrete support to caregivers, such as salary replacement, specialized training, and mental health services, and the original eligibility criteria made it exceedingly difficult for anyone but a spouse to qualify.[14] But while a recent study suggests that there are approximately 627,000 spouses of post–9/11 veterans who do this work, this accounts for only 33 percent of all caregivers for post–9/11 veterans (Ramchand et al. 2014, 29–30, 33). A further 25 percent of caregivers are parents, but almost as many, 23 percent, are categorized as friends and neighbors (34). Since the VA caregiver support program requires caregivers to be either related to or living with the veteran, the vast majority of friends and all neighbors are ineligible for this support. The program also only supports one eligible caregiver at a time, reinforcing the dyadic model of care and undermining the cultivation of more robust caregiving networks, networks that are a fundamental part of the survival strategies in many communities that face ongoing hardship in part because this distribution of care is essential to sustaining care over the long term. There are numerous ways in which the program and its narrow imaginary of family and care fails to offer the kind of support it was designed for. The program may still prove inadequate in cases when arrangement of bodies and affective attachments does conform to that narrow ideal of family and care. Take Rosie, the founder of Burnpits360 mentioned above. She and Leroy are in many ways a model couple for the program. They are a loving couple, and Rosie has committed herself to caring both for Leroy and for the thousands of other veterans who are sick like him. Rosie and Leroy live together, work together, and almost always travel together as nearly all of their many trips across the country are for further testing and treatment for Leroy. Rosie's role as a caregiver is facilitated by the caregiver program, as well, it is worth mentioning, by her decades of experience working in the VA that allows her to navigate its notorious bureaucracy with great skill; her faith in God, which gives her a sense that the compounding vulnerabilities and struggles of her life are for some greater purpose, even if neither she nor Leroy can discern it; and her long-standing propensity for righteous troublemaking. And when she and Leroy travel to Tennessee, Colorado, Utah, or Washington, DC for tests and treatment, the caregiver program offers nothing to help take care of their three children, and no one to keep an eye on Leroy's mother, who lives alone and has dementia and for whom Rosie and Leroy are also responsible. That Rosie and Leroy form not only the idealized caregiving dyad of veteran and wife, but are also parents to three children, caregivers to Leroy's mother, and directors of an advocacy organization that put them both, but especially Rosie, in a position to be supporting many other veterans and caregivers is well beyond the recognition of the family caregiver program, a program designed to stabilize orderly pairs of "significant others."

Among other things, all of this highlights the fact that the picture we have of afterwar work for life is partial, at best. It raises questions about the social forms that such care work does take and should take. Not only might we need to think further about whether the chronic, ongoing, and complex bodily needs of many veterans are best met by spouses, but we might also need to think further about whether any one relationship, or any one person, ought to be doing that work. As in the other facets of war elaborated in this volume, in the case of afterwar work for life, we see the uneven ways the long toll of war is distributed, and the ways that narrow social, cultural, and political imaginaries about who should care and be cared for produce that unevenness giving rise to collateral effects that are felt in the most intimate spaces of domestic life and personal aspiration.

Here are the lessons to be learned from models of improvisational and collective care, especially those that mark themselves as queer or are otherwise intentionally grounded in a political ethics that refuses the normative imperatives of anti-political straight, white, middle-class aspiration and thus diverging from precisely the linking of clinical care and conjugal care that the veteran family caregiver model entails. Such models move beyond thinking of care as a dyadic relationship: They bring broader social and political contexts (such as the nature of community obligation, ethical responsibility, social justice, and the politics of care at multiple levels, from the household to the state) into the practice of care itself, contexts usually identified by scholars of care (Buch 2013; Ehrenreich and Hochschild 2004; Stacey 2011) but not considered as part of the work of care by the people who do it.

To be sure, such models of care still hew closely to bodily need, but they extend thinking about care well beyond diagnostic categories. And, in the way that they put collective practices of care (rather than transactions of caregiving and care-receiving) at the core of a project of conceiving a social world, they might also offer a different way of thinking about suicide. Rather than imagining suicide as the looming threat that the end of a relationship will make real, mobilizing logics of cause and effect and attendant allocations of responsibility, collective practices of care might attend to suicide as a collective and social concern. Rather than a question of the life or death of a body, suicide might appear as a shared experience. Something of the sort seems to be happening in at least one recently publicized case among the marines of the Second Battalion, Seventh Marine Regiment (Phillips 2015). Veterans of this unit, a unit facing a relentless tide of suicides, created a Google spreadsheet with the locations and phone numbers of their comrades so that any one of them in distress could find another nearby and a social media alert system to help identify fellow veterans at risk (ibid.). The arrangement has worked for some. And not for others. But this group of veterans who both struggle with suicide and try to stop others from committing suicide is experimenting with a different mode of care. It is one that is diffuse and whose improvisational and collective nature remaps intimacy, care, and responsibility in ways that extend from the body and beyond the conjugal dyad. Though even here we may find the metaphor of the military family, it is the familiar ethos of military brotherhood, a relation itself historically cross cut with queer intimacies (Serlin 2003), rather than the secluded attachment of the nuclear couple, that animates care.

This is not to say that such models—queer crip care collectives or hybridized online veteran ones—are *the* solution to the problem of veteran need. The clinic and its diagnostic categories and treatments have their important role to play, as does a competent, accountable, and adequately resourced VA. And, in any case, such a "problem" is one that cannot truly be solved as long as there are veterans marked by their experiences of war.[15] But what such models show us is that there are ways of moving beyond the tyranny of the normative ideal of the veteran family caregiver. We might look to them as ways of reimagining both the object of care, and the forms and spaces of sociality and intimacy that make care something that works for life in new ways.

NOTES

1 The most recent annual Disability Statistics Compendium is based on 2017 data and counts 1,662,814 disabled veterans ages 18–64 in the United States (Annual Disability Statistics Compendium 2017). The most recent available numbers from the VA are from 2016 (National Center for Veterans Analysis and Statistics 2018). At that point, they found that 35.9% of all post–9/11 veterans, or roughly 780,000 veterans, had a *documented* service-connected disability, though this is notably lower than the 45% of post–9/11 veterans reported in a 2012 AP story to have *filed* disability claims (Marchione 2012). The Costs of War Project at Brown University's Watson Institute reports that as of January 2015, a minimum of 970,000 post–9/11 veterans have some war-connected disability (www.costsofwar.org).
2 For epidemiological information about post–9/11 veterans treated at VA hospitals, see Office of Public Health 2015.
3 Defense and Veterans Brain Injury Center 2018.
4 I say this mindful of efforts to include the "whole patient" or, more radically, the "whole person" in medical treatment, most notably medical anthropologist Arthur Kleinman's ongoing efforts to humanize medicine. I would suggest such efforts are incredibly important to improving medical care, and there will always be elements of experience that exceed it.
5 Virtually identical charges surface periodically in active duty military contexts, including at the Army's Madigan Healthcare System in 2012 and at Ft. Carson in 2010 and 2015 (Murphy 2012; Zwerdling 2015).
6 Mol (2008), among others, has rightly critiqued the distinction between cure and care at the level of practice, which I also think is essential. I mobilize the distinction here at the level of politics and logics, drawing a distinction between medical trajectories that drive endlessly toward the elimination of a given condition, and those that seek to accommodate it (Clare 2017; see also Kafer 2013, 34–46).
7 Anthropology has showed us time and again, from India (Cohen 2006; Das and Addlakha 2001) to Brazil (Biehl 2005) to Botswana (Livingston 2005), to Chile (Han 2012), to the United States (Heinmann 2015), that the domestic family unit is the normative form of resort for care.
8 Here, I am invoking the work of Elizabeth Povinelli (2006), who gives an account of the conjugal couple as a key transfer point of late liberalism, a social and fleshy configuration that (in its ideal form)—mobilizing ideas of true love and of finding or completing or becoming oneself in it—can peel people away from other unruly intimate configurations and help make them proper liberal subjects.

9 The only notable time it did was when a VA clinician recorded homosexuality as a possible cause of Devin's symptoms in his medical records. Steven wrote enough letters to the right people to have policy implemented that homosexuality could not be recorded in this way in medical records.
10 Written in 1965, *The Negro Family: The Case for National Action* was a report written by then Assistant Secretary of Labor Daniel Patrick Moynihan, intended to highlight the continued effects of the legacies of slavery in African American communities and argue that civil rights legislation had not done enough to address this legacy. However, informed in part by Moynihan's Catholicism, the report argues that African American families are dysfunctional because they are too often female headed, without fathers at home, and characterized by transience, and suggests that the solution to the violent legacy of slavery is not any kind of structural redress, but the disciplining of African American families into heteronormative nuclear households.
11 For a broader discussion of the ecological effects of militarization and war and their implications for health, please see the chapter by Scandlyn and Hautzinger in this volume.
12 In the study, "end of significant relationship" (which is given the normative gloss "loss of significant other") was the most common, and most elaborated, of three "postdeployment stressors" counted. The other two were "financial troubles" and "major life change." The explanation quoted above draws in part on Thomas Joiner's "interpersonal theory of suicide" model which describes three components of suicidal behavior: "thwarted belongingness," "perceived burdensomeness," and "acquired capability" to actually commit the act and experience the associated physical pain.
13 In thinking of care as work for life, I am drawing on Joe Dumit's *Drugs for Life* (2012) and his dual meaning that drugs are "for life, rather than 'for disease,'" and that they are "for life," rather than for a time-limited course.
14 The program was the outcome of the 2010 Omnibus Veterans Healthcare Spending Act and its 2011 extension. The criteria are becoming more flexible as a recognition of the fact that the majority of care work is, in fact, *not* provided by spouses.
15 This fact leads Ken MacLeish (2012) to the haunting observation that suicide is, in a perverse way, a solution of its own.

REFERENCES

Annual Disability Statistics Compendium. 2017. 2017 Annual Report, retrieved from http://disabilitycompendium.org.

Biehl, J. 2005. *Vita: Life in a Zone of Social Abandonment*. Berkeley: University of California Press.

Buch, E. D. 2013. "Senses of Care: Embodying Inequality and Sustaining Personhood in the Home Care of Older Adults in Chicago." *American Ethnologist* 40 (4): 637–650. doi:10.1111/amet.12044.

Chiarelli, P. 2010. *Health Promotion, Risk Reduction, Suicide Prevention*. Washington, DC: US Army.

———. 2012. *Army 2020: Generating Health and Discipline in the Force Ahead of the Strategic Reset*. Washington, DC: US Army.

Chu, D., T. Hall, and S. Jones. 2007. Prepared Statement before the Senate Armed Services Personnel Subcommittee, presented at the Senate Armed Services Personnel Subcommittee, March 28, Washington, DC.

Clare, E. 2017. *Brilliant Imperfection: Grappling with Cure*. Durham, NC: Duke University Press.

Cohen, L. 2006. *No Aging in India: Alzheimer's, the Bad Family, and Other Modern Things*. Berkeley: University of California Press.

Colbert, S. D. 2013. "Black Feminist Collectivity in Ntozake Shange's for Colored Girls Who Have Considered Suicide / When the Rainbow Is Enuf." *Scholar and Feminist Online* 12 (3).

Connell, R. W. 2005. *Masculinities*. Berkeley: University of California Press.

Das, V., and R. Addlakha. 2001. "Disability and Domestic Citizenship: Voice, Gender, and the Making of the Subject." *Public Culture* 13 (3): 511–31.

Defense and Veterans Brain Injury Center. 2018. "DoD Worldwide Numbers for TBI." Retrieved from http://dvbic.dcoe.mil.

Dumit, J. 2012. *Drugs for Life: How Pharmaceutical Companies Define Our Health*. Durham, NC: Duke University Press.

Ehrenreich, B., and A. R. Hochschild, eds. 2004. *Global Woman: Nannies, Maids, and Sex Workers in the New Economy*. New York: Henry Holt.

Foucault, M. 1990. *The History of Sexuality, Vol. 1: An Introduction*. New York: Vintage.

Griffith, J., and M. Vaitkus 2013. "Perspectives on Suicide in the Army National Guard." *Armed Forces and Society* 39 (4): 628–53. doi:10.1177/0095327X12471333.

Han, C. 2012. *Life in Debt: Times of Care and Violence in Neoliberal Chile*. Berkeley: University of California Press.

Heinmann, L. 2015. "Accommodating Care: Transplant Caregiving and the Melding of Health Care with Home Life in the United States." *Medicine Anthropology Theory* 2 (1): 32–56.

Kafer, A. 2013. *Feminist, Queer, Crip*. Bloomington: Indiana University Press.

Kimmel, M. 2006. *Manhood in America: A Cultural History*. Oxford: Oxford University Press.

Kittay, E. 1999. *Love's Labor: Essays on Women, Equality, and Dependency*. New York: Routledge.

Kleinman, A. 2010. "Caregiving: The Divided Meaning of Being Human and the Divided Self of the Caregiver." In *Rethinking the Human*, edited by J. M. Molina and D. K. Swearer. Cambridge, MA: Harvard University Press.

Kristof, N. 2014. "A Loyal Soldier Doesn't Deserve This." *New York Times*, April 13. Retrieved from www.nytimes.com.

Lawrence, Q. 2016. "After Combat Stress, Violence Can Show Up at Home." *All Things Considered*, April 27. Retrieved from www.npr.org.

Livingston, J. 2005. *Debility and Moral Imagination in Botswana*. Bloomington: Indiana University Press.
Lutz, C. 2001. *Homefront: A Military City and the American Twentieth Century*. Boston: Beacon Press.
———. 2013. "US and Coalition Casualties in Iraq and Afghanistan." Retrieved from http://watson.brown.edu/costsofwar.
MacLeish, K. 2012. "Logics of Military Suicide." Paper presented at the Society for Cultural Anthropology, Providence, RI.
———. 2013. *Making War at Fort Hood: Life and Uncertainty in a Military Community*. Princeton, NJ: Princeton University Press.
———. 2018. "On 'Moral Injury': Psychic Fringes and War Violence." *History of the Human Sciences* 31 (2): 128–46.
Marchione, Marilynn. 2012. "Almost Half of Veterans Seek Disability." *Associated Press*, May 27. Retrieved from http://news.yahoo.com.
McArthur, P. 2014. "Sort of Like a Hug: Notes on Collectivity, Conviviality, and Care." *Happy Hypocrite* 7: 48–60.
Mol, A. 2008. *The Logic of Care: Health and the Problem of Patient Choice*. London: Routledge.
Murphy, Kim. 2012. "Army Must Do More to Address Soldiers' Mental Health, Review Says." *Los Angeles Times*, March 8. Retrieved from http://articles.latimes.com.
Office of Public Health. 2015. "VA Health Care Utilization among OEF/OIF/OND Veterans Cumulative from 1st Qtr FY 2002–2nd Qtr FY 2015." Veterans Health Administration. Retrieved from www.publichealth.va.gov.
Oppel Jr., R A., and M. D. Shear. 2014. "Severe Report Finds V.A. Hid Waiting Lists at Hospitals." *New York Times*, May 28. Retrieved from www.nytimes.com.
Phillips, D. 2015. "In Unit Stalked by Suicide, Veterans Try to Save One Another." *New York Times*, September 20. Retrieved from www.nytimes.com.
Povinelli, E. 2006. *The Empire of Love*. Durham, NC: Duke University Press.
Ramchand, R., T. L. Tanielian, M. P. Fisher, C. A. Vaughan, and T. E. Trail. 2014. *Hidden Heroes: America's Military Caregivers*. Santa Monica, CA: Rand Corporation.
Russ, A. J. 2005. "Love's Labor Paid For: Gift and Commodity at the Threshold of Death." *Cultural Anthropology* 20 (1): 128–55.
Serlin, D. H. 2003. "Crippling Masculinity: Queerness and Disability in U.S. Military Culture, 1800–1945." *GLQ: A Journal of Lesbian and Gay Studies* 9 (1): 149–79.
Shuttleworth, R., N. Wedgwood, and N. J. Wilson. 2012. "The Dilemma of Disabled Masculinity." *Men and Masculinities* 15 (2): 174–94. doi:10.1177/1097184X12439879.
Stacey, C. L. 2011. *The Caring Self: The Work Experiences of Home Care Aides*. Ithaca, NY: Cornell University Press.
Terry, J. 2017. *Attachments to War*. Durham, NC: Duke University Press.
US Department of Veterans Affairs. VA Caregiver Support. Diagnosis Care Sheets. Retrieved from www.caregiver.va.gov.
Watson, E., and M. E. Shaw, eds. 2011. *Performing American Masculinities: The 21st-Century Man in Popular Culture*. Bloomington: Indiana University Press.

Wood, D. 2012. "Beyond the Battlefield: Afghanistan's Wounded Struggle with Genital Injuries." *Huffington Post*, March 21. Retrieved from www.huffingtonpost.com.

Wool, Z. H. 2013. "On Movement: The Matter of Soldiers' Bodies After Combat." *Ethnos* 78 (3): 403–33.

———. 2015. *After War: The Weight of Life at Walter Reed*. Durham, NC: Duke University Press.

———. 2016. "Attachments of Life: Intimacy, Genital Injury, and the Flesh of the U.S. Soldier Body." In *Living and Dying in the Contemporary World: A Compendium*, edited by V. Das and C. Han, 399–417. Oakland: University of California Press.

Wool, Z. H., and S. Messinger. 2012. "Labors of Love: The Transformation of Care in the Non-Medical Attendant Program at Walter Reed Army Medical Center." *Medical Anthropology Quarterly* 26 (1): 26–48.

Zwerdling, Daniel. 2015. "Thousands of Soldiers with Mental Health Disorders Kicked Out for 'Misconduct.'" *National Public Radio*, October 28.

11

"It's Not Okay"

War's Toll on Health Brought Home to Communities and Environments

JEAN SCANDLYN AND SARAH HAUTZINGER

In a room full of veterans, family members, service providers, and activists, Dolores, a young wife of an infantry sergeant, thanked everyone for the opportunity to "bring up awareness of our real lives, behind closed doors." Her husband joined the army to fulfill his dream of becoming a command sergeant major. His first deployment was to Iraq, with a unit that would stand out for post-deployment troubles. "You know, a lot of my husband's soldiers are in jail. . . . There's a lot of murders, a lot of domestic violence. A lot of them are part of his unit." After that first deployment, she said, her husband self-medicated with alcohol. During his second tour to Iraq in 2006, he suffered a traumatic brain injury (TBI) following a blast from an improvised explosive device (IED). It was after this deployment that Dolores noticed significant changes in his behavior. She urged him to seek help at Fort Carson, which he did, only to be turned away by an army doctor who said, "There's nothing wrong with you. You're faking it." Dolores went to see the physician, who agreed to diagnose her husband with PTSD (posttraumatic stress disorder) and submit papers for a medical discharge. "How am I supposed to help him get to where he was before without any help, without any knowledge? You know the military didn't tell us about PTSD. They didn't tell us about traumatic brain injury. They didn't tell us that they were going to come back different." Dolores began to cry. She said she didn't know how to answer her children when they said, "I want my old daddy back." War exacts costs not only where battles are fought, but in the communities where soldiers prepare for war, and to which they return.

In the six years since her husband's return, Dolores quit her job to provide and advocate for his care. She told of how her husband still feels responsible for helping out soldiers from his unit who are suffering from PTSD and other effects of the war to the extent that she felt he was neglecting his own family and their needs. She spoke of her children's grades falling and their having emotional problems requiring mental health services. She ended her talk, "It's not ok. It's not ok. It's not ok."

Dolores's story illustrates the myriad ways that war affects everyone—civilian and military personnel and institutions at home as well as abroad. Many who shared their experiences with us, as anthropologists studying army veterans and their families in Colorado Springs, Colorado, understood themselves as deeply entangled in the Iraq and Afghanistan wars. Assessing war's toll on health requires that we consider the ways we all become entangled in wars seemingly distant, and how war particularly erodes wellness in domestic military communities. Colorado Springs, Colorado, is home to the US Air Force Academy, Peterson and Schriever air force bases, NORAD (North American Aerospace Defense Command), and Fort Carson, one of the largest and most active army bases in the United States that sent many tens of thousands of soldiers to Iraq and Afghanistan in the dozen years from 2003 to 2015. We focus not primarily on active-duty soldiers or on their physical wounds, but on how militarization affects the health of soldiers and their families, extending to the communities in which they live.[1]

Holistic and comprehensive conceptions of health are defined to include "physical, mental, and social well-being, and not merely the absence of disease or infirmity" (World Health Organization 1948). Although the WHO adopted this definition of health immediately after World War II, during the postwar era, it was largely eclipsed by a biomedical model focused on the cure and eradication of diseases in individuals through medical technology and individual behavior change (Birn, Pillay, and Holtz 2009; Farmer et al. 2006). Neoliberal approaches to economic development in the 1980s and 1990s infused public health as well, furthering the biomedical approach to health (Farmer 2005; Hahn 1999; Birn et al. 2009). In the past decade, as HIV and other infectious diseases have emerged or "re-emerged" (Farmer 1999), a holistic definition of health has also "re-emerged," one that recognizes social, political, economic, and environmental factors as the *actual* determinants of health (Berkman and Kawachi 2014; Krieger 1994). Using this model to understand the costs of war on human health, alongside recognition of war-related mental and physical injuries to individuals, we must consider issues like employment, income and debt, education, family dynamics and stresses, social cohesion, and community safety. The stories of individuals and families affected by war reveal this best, and importantly, go beyond the effects on individuals to demonstrate the effects of war on population health as reflected in challenges faced by community organizations and institutions.

From 2008 to 2014, we led a team of undergraduate and graduate students who studied the effects of war on military personnel, their families, and the community of Colorado Springs. We began by interviewing active-duty soldiers in an infantry battalion that had recently returned from a harrowing tour of duty in Iraq and was preparing for another tour in Afghanistan. But we quickly realized that to understand more comprehensively the effects of war on health, we had to talk to family members, healthcare providers, leaders of civic organizations serving military personnel and veterans, and members of the community who became the first responders to soldiers returning with PTSD, TBI, substance abuse and other risky behaviors, anger and violence, suicidality, and depression. We attended military-civilian town hall–style meetings, resilience training, reintegration sessions, and healing sessions that implemented everything from work with horses in a corral to varied shamanic approaches—Lakota- and Hopi-based sweat lodges, or soul retrievals based in guided visualization.

Because we followed soldiers to their mental health and social service providers at Fort Carson, and later to the homes, family members, and communities to which they returned, our findings reflect the current values and cultural norms of US military institutions. There are, however, important changes afoot. When we began our research in 2008, "Don't Ask, Don't Tell" was still in effect. Whereas military social service and mental health providers at Fort Carson might work with single-parent families, divorced parents with joint custody of children, female soldiers married to male civilians, and gay families on an individual basis, group-based programs still assumed a heterosexual norm, which our material in turn reflects. Written materials referred to Army Spouses, capitalized, and those in domestic unions or partnerships, regardless of their sexual identity or orientation, had little recognition and few rights. If soldiers were not legally married, which at the time largely precluded those in marriages with same-sex or trans partners, they could not list their spouse or partner as next of kin to receive notice of serious injury or death. While we did interview a few soldiers who openly identified as queer, we did not collect sufficient data to speak to the effects of war on health that are specific to individuals who identify as LGBTQ, their partners, and families. Only recently have researchers studied the health of these individuals and families (for recent research on this topic, see Zoë Wool's chapter in this volume; Goldbach and Castro 2016; Brown and Jones 2015; Burks 2011; Biddix, Fogel, and Black 2013; Katz 2010).

War and the Health of Families

A deployment occurs when the military sends personnel and material from their home base to another location, usually to a site of conflict. For service members and their families, deployments are more than military actions: They bring a host of practical and emotional issues for those at home. Dolores's repetition—"It's not okay"—highlights three major ways in which war affects the health of families: It affects children, the spouse who remains at home, and marital or other intimate partner relationships.

For children, a parent's deployment means that person is absent from home for days, months, or years in a setting that older children learn to associate with the risk of bodily harm or death. The majority of parents we interviewed worked hard to minimize the disruption and distress to their children's lives. Some emphasized maintaining family traditions and daily routines, while others moved to be close to extended family members who could provide support for the parent staying at home. Nonetheless, deployment can be a time of marked stress for children, with their responses to that stress varying by age and developmental stage, the number of parents' deployments, and across all stages of the deployment cycle (Lester et al. 2010).

While very young children may not understand the risks their deployed parent faces, the parent at home and older siblings are aware of these dangers and may communicate their concern and fear to the young child. Young children's health is strongly determined by their parents' health and well-being. As a consequence, a parent's depression and anxiety during and after deployments, especially that of the parent at home caring for children, is highly associated with their children's mental health as measured in levels of anxiety, acting out, and depression (Flake et al. 2009; Lester et al. 2010). Young children with deployed parents see pediatricians more frequently for mental and behavioral health issues than those whose parents are not deployed (Gorman, Eide, and Hisle-Gorman 2010; Chartrand et al. 2008). Mental health providers we interviewed spoke of "very, very explosive and aggressive" behavior and decreased scores on measures of resilience in preschool age children with deployed parents. A Head Start teacher we spoke with worried about depression-related aggression and suicidality in her young charges.

Older children and girls of all ages have more problems with school, family, and peer relationships when a parent deploys (Chandra et al. 2009), while younger children and boys, on the other hand, are at higher risk for depressive and behavioral symptoms (Cozza et al. 2010). Laurie Wilson is the principal of Milton High School, an alternative high school for at-risk students, where half of the students come from military families. Wilson says that adolescents learning new roles in the family when a parent deploys may experience high levels of stress, a pattern identified in several studies of adolescents in military families (Knobloch et al. 2015; Esposito-Smythers et al. 2011). "Whether they're stepping in as Dad or whether they're stepping in as Mom . . . having to get a job, or having to become babysitters to the brothers and sisters. Or they're taking on extra responsibilities at home. And that cuts into their school time, whether it's attending school or doing their [home]work."

Such pressures are not unusual for children with working parents, but they weigh more heavily and take on different meanings in the context of repeated deployments. Students often miss school to spend time with a parent who is about to deploy, who is home on mid-tour leave, or to prepare for their homecoming. Stress often manifests in behavioral problems. According to Kathy Edwards, the children's program manager at a Colorado Springs agency that provides services to victims of sexual abuse and assault, when a parent deploys, children "can't emotionally regulate so they're having significant behavior problems, they're having significant academic problems in school, they're having problems with their relationships with peers—they're fighting because they have this overwhelming fear." Huebner et al. (2007) found that the ambiguity of loss when parents deployed was a significant source of stress and changes in mental health in adolescents.

At times the depression is severe enough to require professional help or hospitalization (Esposito-Smythers et al. 2011). Worrying about their deployed parent's safety can make concentrating on schoolwork difficult, and students' academic performance may suffer, with possible long-term consequences if they fall behind (Engel, Gallagher, and Lyle 2010; Flake et al. 2009). In contrast, focusing on school activities and peer relationships can distract from the fear. And adolescents from military families may view taking on new responsibilities and having a parent who is serving in the military as sources of pride, new skills, self-confidence, and independence (NMFA 2008; Huebner and Mancini 2005).

Deployments can also affect spouses' mental and physical health. Deployments of nine months or longer and more frequent deployments place female spouses at greater risk for depression, anxiety, and sleep disorders (Mansfield et al. 2010; Sherman and Bowling 2011; Allen et al. 2011; Lester et al. 2010). As JJ, one of the spouse-mothers we interviewed, described it, "You cry, you know, when you have to. And you try not to worry about it. My whole philosophy is you've got little kids—don't be cryin' every single minute of the day and freakin' them out, you know. It's all about how mommy handles it, and how the kids are going to handle it." According to Kathy Edwards, mentioned above, if a mother is not used to being a single parent and is overwhelmed herself, she may be unable to "create the safety, stability, security they need. Mom's stressed, overburdened, can't emotionally regulate herself." Edwards reports high levels of child abuse during deployment as a consequence.

Cynthia Enloe has pointed out that part of the agreement a woman may make in service to playing the role of the "Good Military Wife" includes prioritizing her husband's performance as the measure of her family's well-being, being a competent single parent managing household finances and chores, being "pleased to relinquish" head-of-household duties on his return, and tolerating the results of his deployment stress, "liking moving" (changing where the family is stationed) and viewing it as an exciting opportunity, enjoying unpaid work, and taking pride at her own children entering the military (Enloe 2000, 162–164). Even before the 9/11 wars, wives' clubs or family support groups "once fully staffed by Army-wife volunteers and regarded as 'nice to have' were now recognized as critical to Army life" (Keller 2006, xxix). Such recognition led to a concerted effort by the army to bring Family Readiness Groups' unpaid, support work increasingly "under the chain of command" through the early 2000s (USAWC 2009; Hautzinger and Scandlyn 2014, 145–146). Folding FRGs into the command structure has had multiple effects; while it enables more reliable support and can prevent spouses and families (especially those of junior enlisted soldiers) from falling through the cracks, it can also undercut spousal autonomy and FRG involvement as largely social, bringing it closer, for some, to "mandatory fun" for which spouses may feel "volunTOLD." Regardless, the "force multiplying" effects are unmistakable: Family stability supports soldier readiness and deployability.

Running a household, advancing a career, and raising children as a single parent, military or civilian, can be overwhelming and lonely. Despite her strong self-assurance, JJ acknowledged that handling deployments wasn't always easy. "The first deployment to Iraq was hard. The kids were little, two and five. We had just moved back here. I really didn't know a whole lot of people at first, and it was scary because it was right after 9/11. Everybody was just afraid." During one of her husband's deployments, JJ was very active with her Family Readiness Group. Through her work, JJ observed many young wives who were not coping well, feeling overwhelmed parenting young children on their own, lacking the skills to manage a household budget and either running out of money or going into debt buying on installment plans. She observed women who took up with other men while their husbands were in Iraq or Afghanistan.

Because we worked with an infantry battalion, which at the time had only seven women, our information was gleaned primarily from female spouses. Male spouses, or "MANspouses," as one blogger called himself, are increasing in numbers but are still largely invisible. Little is expected of male spouses in terms of participating in official activities like the Family Readiness Group (Gassmann 2010). In fact, female spouses may actively discourage their participation (Hautzinger and Scandlyn 2014, 160–164).

The US military is a socially conservative organization. Although people who identify as LGBTQ may now serve openly in the military, and women may now serve in all military occupational specialties including combat roles, strictly normative gendered roles and practices still infuse military institutions, with roles identified with masculine traits more highly valued. For example, front-line, infantry ground troops may be maligned as "grunts" and "cannon fodder," but they are also viewed as "real soldiers," formerly "real men," the "tip of the spear," that penetrates enemy lines. Soldiers who work in support roles as clerks with office jobs on the relatively more protected bases are "fobbits," a combination of "Forward Operating Base" or "FOB" and the home-loving, short-statured hobbits of J.R.R. Tolkien (1997). A Google search for images of fobbits reveals the gendered stereotypes and negative judgments of those who play supportive roles to the masculine—whether male or female—front-line soldier.

Women and mothers who themselves deploy face challenges, including danger and risk to their own health and well-being (Naclerio 2015), arranging supervision and custody of children when they are deployed, facing children who don't recognize them after a year-long absence, and self- and social judgment by civilians who find it hard to understand how a mother could leave her children (Thorpe 2014). Jessica Scott, a first lieutenant in the army, tells of women who lost custody of their children while deployed, with one lawyer arguing that "leaving her children for military service is no way for a mother to act" (Scott 2010; Weinstein and White 1997; Waterston 2009).

Many marriages cannot survive the stress of long and multiple deployments. For all military personnel who entered military service and married in the military from March 1999 to June 2008, the greater the number of months of deployment the higher the risk of divorce, with 97 percent of the divorces in this group occurring after return from a deployment (Negrusa, Negrusa, and Hosek 2014). "Divorce rates are higher among both combat soldiers and veterans" (Burland and Lundquist 2013, 16, 17).

Divorce can hold dire health consequences among veterans. Dissolution of a marriage or romantic relationship is one of the chief life events associated with veterans' committing suicide (Gottman, Gottman, and Atkins 2011; Lusk et al. 2015). While this may suggest that war is not the primary factor in military suicides, we argue that the rising divorce rate among military personnel is itself an expression of the toll of militarization more generally. The separation of deployment coupled with the dangers of being in theater contribute to poor communication and conflict among spouses and high levels of perceived emotional betrayal (Gottman et al. 2011).

Reintegration and PTSD

As another way in which our society reduces the effects of militarization to problems at the individual and family level, PTSD, a psychological condition resulting from exposure to life-threatening trauma, has dominated public conversations and media treatment of the effects of the wars in Iraq and Afghanistan on US military personnel. But PTSD alone fails to capture the many effects of war on families and communities that cannot be explained by mental illness alone or at all. One way to recognize these broader effects is to focus on soldiers' reintegration into civilian life.

Beneath the music, the flags, the speeches and prayers, the tears and ecstatic embraces of soldiers' homecoming from war also lie ambivalence and anxiety. Many soldiers simply want to get home. Other soldiers scan the crowds searching for someone they expected to greet them who has not shown up. Children may be seeing a parent they barely remember. Spouses may wonder how they are going to establish intimacy after a year of tightly controlled communication (around limited time, technology, and topics, while maintaining upbeat tones) and renegotiate responsibilities in light of new roles they have assumed (Booth, Segal, and Bell 2007, 42).

As Theresa, who is married to a special operations soldier said,

> I've gotten a new husband three different times. So much changes . . . If you're interrogating and working in the community [in Iraq] trying to find people you have to learn how to completely compartmentalize everything, you can't have emotions. Coming home, you have to turn that off and sometimes it takes a while. Sometimes it's hard to remember his kids are his kids and you're allowed to have emotion.

As soldiers make the transition home, they may be "ambiguously present," that is, they are present physically but absent psychologically (Faber et al. 2008), preoccupied with relationships with fellow soldiers formed during deployment, losses of comrades who died or were severely injured, and changes in the intensity and structure of their work that may leave them feeling aimless/purposeless and unsure of how to act. Distance from the war zone may create space for soldiers, now veterans, to reflect on their experiences and question their own actions and those of others (Gutmann and Lutz 2010).

These questions and the memories that generate them may be a human response to the challenges war presents to core values and not necessarily indications of PTSD or major depression. Veterans may experience anxiety, anger, shame, grief, and sadness that contribute to feeling out of control (Maguen and Litz 2012, 1). Such symptoms may reflect moral injury, defined as "perpetrating, failing to prevent, bearing witness to, or learning about acts that transgress deeply held moral beliefs and expectations" (Litz et al. 2009).

Compounding war-related sources of distress may be financial problems incurred during deployments or the loss of combat pay. Financial distress is another risk factor for suicide, relationship problems, and depression (Black, Gallaway, and Ritchie 2011). Discharge from the military presents its own challenges. For many young recruits, like this one we spoke with, this may be the first time they have lived as adults and civilians.

> We are completely institutionalized. I hate that word, but it's true. We don't know how to make small talk or dress for a job interview—soldiers need a fashion show. We think sergeant is a first name! We've been told what to wear, what to do, what to think, every day for years. We need help coming back in.

Veterans must move from a world where they made few personal decisions to one filled with constant choices and alternatives, where they must create their own structure and find their own meaning and purpose. Further complicating this process is frequent alienation, and even contempt for, civilian "culture" inculcated in many military circles.

Thus, even in the absence of PTSD, major depression, traumatic brain injury, or a visible physical wound, war takes a toll that may only be realized during reintegration. Kenneth MacLeish (2013) documents the wear and tear on young, healthy bodies resulting from carrying heavy loads of weapons and protective gear in harsh conditions, wear and tear that soldiers are trained to deny and bear. As a consequence, many soldiers or their health providers do not acknowledge these stress-related physical injuries as service-related disabilities, and service members are denied appropriate healthcare and rehabilitation and are uncompensated for loss of livelihood.

Returning veterans suffering from mental illness may face a serious dearth of accessible services. Considering mental health care services alone, Colorado ranks thirty-second nationally for publicly funded mental health care, leaving many residents, especially those like veterans, with serious and complex mental illness or those living in rural areas of the state, without adequate care (TriWest Group 2011). Although active-duty military personnel and their family members can receive mental health care through TriCARE, the military's health insurance program, and qualifying veterans through the Veterans Administration, many prefer care from community-based civilian providers, and Fort Carson's mental health services are themselves chronically understaffed (Hautzinger and Scandlyn 2014).

Soldiers may seek relief for pain and emotional distress by using drugs and alcohol (Ramchard et al. 2011; Wilk et al. 2010; Mash et al. 2014). They may also act out in violent ways—in barroom brawls, through child abuse, and through attacks on their spouses and partners (Marshall, Panuzio, and Taft 2005), although the relationship between anger and hostility in Iraq and Afghanistan war veterans is complex and not well understood (Elbogen et al. 2010; Killgore et al. 2008). As veteran Ronald Rhuesenburg described, "My heart starts beating really fast. If someone just shuts the door really quick, you know, that gets me. My patience has gone down a lot for a lot of stupid stuff. But to me, it is not noticeable. Some guys have a lot more issues with it, with their attitude. They're always angry and have drinking problems." Whereas unintentional injuries are the number one cause of death in US males ages 20–34 and in Colorado (CDC 2015), there is some evidence that risk-taking is more common among veterans returning from combat (Killgore et al. 2008).

Many soldiers told us of the addiction to the "high" and "adrenalin rush" of combat that they seek when they return home by engaging in high-risk activities like riding motorcycles or bungee- and base jumping. Especially when coupled with alcohol use, these activities may result in disabling and fatal injuries (Moore 2015). Fort Carson has an active injury prevention program and requires soldiers to take a course in motorcycle operation and safety and to wear helmets if they ride on the post. As you exit Fort Carson from the main gate, there is a large sign proclaiming how many days the post has been free of fatal traffic crashes.

Sarah Jones, a counselor who assists victims of domestic violence in Colorado Springs, noticed a distinctive pattern in domestic violence following deployments. "When they returned, rates were pretty average, maybe even a little lower for the first 30 [days], normal at 60 and doubled at 90." She explained that symptoms of combat-related PTSD and depression may not appear immediately following return from a combat zone: "It takes two or three months before the depression sets in." This delay in reporting symptoms upon return from deployment is well documented. Proposed reasons for the delay include relief at returning to the United States and reluctance to delay going on post-deployment leave if they report symptoms requiring further assessment or treatment (Bliese et al. 2007). Counselors at Fort Carson noted that the early days and weeks following return from deployment represent a "honeymoon" period in which the excitement of reunion may overshadow conflicts that later emerge related to the symptoms of PTSD, depression, or traumatic brain injury.

Community Health

Violence may spill out into the community. As we began our research, officers of the 2–12 Battalion, recently returned from a second tour to Iraq and preparing for a first tour to Afghanistan, struggled to confront psychological and behavioral issues—increasing rates of PTSD, depression and other diagnoses, suicide (Blumenthal 2012 and 2017), violence and criminality—all of which represented relatively new territory for which they had little expertise. Between 2006 and 2008, soldiers, most of them from the 2–12, were responsible for fourteen murders in Colorado Springs (Hautzinger and Scandlyn 2014, 73–95).

Problematic behavior is often the first and only way that veterans obtain professional help. Soldier Daniel Quest described a "buddy" who saw his best friend "killed right in front of him." The soldier snapped, and since that time,

> He's had all sorts of run-ins with the law. Since he's been back, he's lost like half of his pay because he's always getting in trouble for something. It's just ridiculous. He needs help and he's starting to get it now, but it took him shooting a gun off in public for him to get the help. He was downtown at the club. He took the gun away from somebody else and held him at gunpoint and discharged the weapon in the air.

The Veterans Trauma Court in Colorado Springs is a direct response to veterans with alcohol- or drug-related charges and charges of public and domestic violence. Recognizing that many of these veterans suffer from PTSD, TBI, and depression, the court uses a restorative justice model to mandate actions that directly address the symptoms of acting out as well as the veteran's psychiatric illness. Even in the model VTC courtroom, we felt an air of heaviness, as we watched veterans struggle against pain, frustration, and the near futility of sharing their stories, given the breadth and magnitude of the challenges they faced. Each of the VTC program participants searches for a path out of their own particular labyrinth of financial, social, and health-related problems. They went from having had full-time (military) jobs with benefits and the camaraderie of military service to being caught in a relentless spiral of court hearings, indebtedness, unemployment, and often homelessness.

The effects of violence on the community are not restricted to the acts of a few veterans. The majority of veterans and those with PTSD do not commit violent crimes; however, these murders and spikes in child abuse and domestic violence among military personnel are part of the more general social and cultural effects of militarization in the United States. War permits the use of lethal force to kill and wound, which goes against our peacetime socialization to protect life. War supports the idea that some, if not many, social problems can only be solved through violence. A comparative study by Dane Archer and Rosemary Gartner (1976) found that homicide rates increased significantly and pervasively (and not just among veterans) following wars spanning from World War I through Vietnam.

The all-volunteer force (AVF), instituted after the draft was dissolved in 1973, has affected community health in several ways. It has concentrated military service among families in rural areas of the country, particularly in the Southeast and Southwest, with a tradition of military service and limited or shrinking economic opportunities. This has created a "casualty gap" between rich and poor communities that bear the burden of caring for disabled veterans and the deaths of their young people (Kriner and Shen 2010). The relatively small size of the AVF—less than 1 percent of the national population—has contributed to a "military-civilian gap" that often leaves civilians and veterans feeling isolated from one another and unsure of how to reach out to offer or accept support and assistance.

Examining what preparing for war demands not only of individuals, but also of their communities and surrounding landscapes, demonstrates the diverse dimensions through which war is, inevitably, brought home and then continues to take a health toll on communities.

Preparing for War: Ecology and Health

War is "brought home" from afar, with pasts sustained through traumatic memory, in terms that are predominantly emotional and psychological. Yet far earlier in the production cycle, as prelude to its exportation, domestic preparation for war inflicts ecological injuries, with immediate implications for health.

Of 1,300 Superfund sites in the United States, fully 900 are abandoned military facilities or sites involved with the manufacture or testing of military materials (Reuben 2010, 77). Sciencecorps, a group of physicians concerned that veterans understand the "potential health effects they may experience due to chemical exposure during military service" (2012), identified seven categories of hazardous chemicals commonly used on air bases, many of which are also present on other military bases. These include: solvents, petroleum fuels, pesticides, toxic heavy metals, radioactive materials, asbestos and other fibers, and engine maintenance products. Exposure to these chemicals can damage kidneys, lungs, the liver, eyes, and the nervous system, and cause birth defects, cancer, and cardiac arrhythmias. Many of these effects first appear long after people leave the military, but unless exposure is clearly documented during service, veterans have little basis on which to claim treatment or disability benefits.

The chemicals used on military bases can leach into surrounding communities' land and water, though systematic research has been hampered by the Department of Defense's resistance to outside scrutiny (Hynes 2011). For example, exposure to solvents benzene and trichloroethylene (TCE) used at Camp LeJeune in North Carolina and present in the surrounding community's water supply were associated with neural tube defects in infants whose mothers consumed the water during the first trimester of pregnancy (Ruckart, Bove, and Maslia 2013). Residents of Vieques, Puerto Rico, the site of a naval training base, had a rate of cancer twice as high as the rest of the island, high rates of early sexual development in girls, and a high incidence of potentially pathological changes in heart muscles from low-frequency noise.

In Colorado, the military's activities have had a large environmental impact. Just 70 miles north of Colorado Springs, adjacent to Denver, the Army Corps of Engineers declared Rocky Mountain Arsenal, where the army stored toxic wastes in the decades between World War II and the Vietnam War, "the earth's most toxic square mile" (Hynes 2011). More recently, in suburbs south of Colorado Springs, the Air Force has assumed responsibility for water and soil contamination caused by use of a firefighting foam with toxic perfluorinated chemicals at a thousand times permitted levels and tied to low birth weights; these effects had been known for more than thirty years (Finley 2017). Two Fort Carson training-exercise fires in 2018, together covering more than 600 acres and forcing hundreds of civilian evacuations, were contained only after burning for a six-week period (Forster 2018).

The wars in Iraq and Afghanistan have contributed to the expansion of the Piñon Canyon Maneuver Site (PCMS) in southeastern Colorado (Hautzinger and Scandlyn 2014, 197–201). In 1983, the Department of Defense obtained the current parcel of land for the PCMS, through the largest condemnation of lands in US history. In 2004, a report entitled "Piñon Vision" revealed plans to gradually increase military holdings to 6.9 *million* acres—nearly a quarter of the state of Colorado—across five phases, making the PCMS three times larger than any other military base in the United States. Creating the "Pentagon's 51st state," as some call it (Vatic Project 2011), would displace 17,000 residents. On terrain so delicate that Santa Fe Trail wheel ruts are still visible, 67-ton Abrams tanks and 18-ton Stryker combat vehicles do worse, along with live-fire exercises—in a place where lightning sparks grass fires that burn hundreds of acres at a go. When soldiers were leaving Fort Carson for Iraq, the army built mock Iraqi villages; when deployments moved to Afghanistan, the army emphasized Colorado's high altitude and PCMS's proximity to the mountains for flight-based training and brought a helicopter-based brigade to the region (CSAction 2011).

In light of the ongoing public outcry about water, and noise and air pollution linked to southern Colorado as a launching pad for military deployment, we observe that war presents risks and harm to human health and well-being prior to, and geographically distant from, the locations where battles are fought, including the wider communities near military bases.

War, Militarization, and Health

Militarization affects not only military personnel or people working under contract to the military contractors, but every citizen (Lutz and Millar 2012; Gonzalez 2010; Enloe 2007, 2010). It affects individual health when veterans are unemployed and homeless or land in jail from substance use; or when a spouse must quit her job to care for a disabled veteran; or a teenager is hospitalized for depression during a parent's deployment. It affects a community's health when bodies are damaged by toxic wastes left from firing ranges and other military activities; when ill health effects follow from noise and air pollution resulting from helicopter training missions; when police and social services are stretched to handle barroom brawls among returning service members or to aiding homeless veterans; or when communities lose land to military expansion that could be used for ranching or recreation.

Philosopher Elaine Scarry states what should be obvious: "The main purpose and outcome of war is injuring" (1985, 63). Battle monuments and war memorials, like the ring of sandstone slabs at Fort Caron that list the names of soldiers killed in battle or as a result of their wounds, are a visible reminder of war's toll on human health. Zoë Wool, in this volume and in her book *After War* (2015), documents the injuries war inflicts, and the scars it leaves behind both on veterans and those who care for them. Nor are the costs of war evenly distributed across the population. The highest proportion of war deaths falls on communities already burdened by poverty, low levels of education, and few economic opportunities (Kriner and Shen 2010). Our work (Hautzinger and Scandlyn 2014) and that of Erin Finley (2011) illustrate war's mental injuries in PTSD, major depression, and traumatic brain injury. These injuries, too, create scars that may cause pain and suffering decades after combat ends. Soldiers bring these injuries home to their living rooms and communities, compounding what "collateral damage," from conflicts at thousands of miles' distance, can mean.

In many respects, American society does recognize war's damage to health by providing death benefits to widows/-ers and orphans, and compensation and benefits to injured veterans. It is undeniable that such benefits often fall far short of need or are administered under bureaucratic rules that lack the timeliness or flexibility that veterans and those who care for them need to arrange and pay for short- and long-term care. And, by emphasizing and even *requiring* disability and pathology, benefits can create long-term dependence that can interfere with healing and recovery.

As Dolores said in this chapter's opening, "It's not ok." Even adequate treatment of the visible physical wounds and readily detectable mental wounds is simply not enough. If we define health holistically, if we recognize connection to others as a foundation of individual health, if we embrace the social conditions of life as the actual determinants of health, then to promote and protect health, we must consider all of war's effects and take responsibility for its true costs.

What does this mean? Above all, it means understanding the occupational hazards of military work beyond the dangers of combat. As Ken MacLeish has shown in *Making War at Fort Hood* (2013), soldiers may be at the peak of physical fitness, but they must carry heavy equipment and protective gear that can result in lifelong orthopedic problems and pain. Despite the integration of women into all military roles and the repeal of "Don't Ask, Don't Tell," the military is still a highly socially and culturally conservative institution in which enlisted personnel and officers alike use strongly differentiated masculine and feminine norms—and often of markedly misogynistic or homophobic bents—to enforce conformity and motivate behavior. This affects not only behavior, but how military personnel evaluate their worth and the value of their service. And it shows up in the high rates of sexual assault and rape in the military that may create long-term difficulties in establishing intimacy. Because of the residual effects of Don't Ask, Don't Tell, we may not know for some time to come, if ever, the full extent of sexual assault on individuals who identify as LGBTQ.

While we understand the devastation soldiers face if they lose a limb, or if a "battle buddy" dies, we may not recognize the losses that are suffered when soldiers return home or leave the military, how these can affect health over the long term, and how they tax collective networks. Literally, this means adding cost columns when we calculate the benefits of military funds, and figuratively, it means remembering that this is an economy based on injury and death. It means understanding how military institutions may make marriage and childbearing at younger ages possible for low-income young people, but also subject those young marriages to repeated separations that may drive couples apart, amplifying depression and suicidality. Military wages can support a family, but in the lower ranks still may not be enough to live debt-free. Financial stress can increase conflict in relationships and contribute to depression and suicide. The military brings people together for long periods of time, but that intimacy often dissipates, or may be hard to replace, in civilian life—again, making readjustment to civilian life difficult, and contributing to depression and isolation. Rates of binge drinking are higher among young adults in the military than their civilian counterparts, and rates of substance use are also high. Substance and alcohol use, in turn, are associated with intimate partner violence, child abuse, fighting, arrests, unemployment, and homelessness. Whereas these effects of war may be recognized in communities with a large military presence like Colorado Springs, which has an extensive network of service providers and organizations dedicated to serving veterans and their families, support and assistance may be harder to access for veterans and reservists living in rural communities.

It is important, finally, to acknowledge that aspects of military culture can promote health: For example, military communities are notable for distinctive levels of physical fitness, for observation of high standards of hygiene and order, for teamwork and mutual care within communities, and for the development of response skills in the face of emergencies and other difficult situations. The sense of purpose, and of dedication to a mission greater than oneself, is something many veterans find lacking in civilian life, which often makes their adjustment difficult. Decoupling these positive, health-promoting aspects of military life from their association with the negative effects of state-sanctioned violence on domestic and civilian life could help us understand and assess more fully the costs of war.[2]

The labyrinthine entanglements of war, across vast distances and highly variable social, psychological, and ecological dimensions, augurs to the persistent veiling and underestimation of its costs on health and wholeness. From the Rocky Mountain West's state of Colorado, where much of the direct and indirect morbidity and mortality of the post–9/11 wars remain distant, the imprint of the "syndemics of war" (Ostrach and Singer 2013), and the synergistic interactions of war-related devastation, nonetheless ring loud and clear.

NOTES

This chapter is adapted from *Beyond Post-Traumatic Stress: Homefront Struggles with the Wars on Terror* (Hautzinger and Scandlyn 2014). We are grateful to the publisher, Left Coast Press (now Routledge), for permission to reprint portions of the original text here.

1 For a discussion of wounded soldiers and veterans and the effects on their families, see Finley 2011 and Wool 2015.
2 Outward Bound is a good example. Based on a training program for British seamen to improve survival rates after World War II, Outward Bound became a model for experiential learning. Many US corporations use Outward Bound as part of their leadership training programs.

REFERENCES

Allen, E. S., G. K. Rhoades, S. M. Stanly, and H. J. Markman. 2011. "On the Home Front: Stress for Recently Deployed Army Couples." *Family Process* 50(2): 235–247.

Archer, D., and R. Gartner. 1976. "Violent Acts and Violent Times: A Comparative Approach to Postwar Homicide Rates." *American Sociological Review* 41(6): 937–963.

Berkman, L. F., and I. Kawachi. 2014. A Historical Framework for Social Epidemiology: Social Determinants of Population Health." In L. F. Berkman, I. Kawachi, and M. M. Glymour (Eds.), *Social Epidemiology* (pp. 1–16). Oxford: Oxford University Press.

Biddix, J. M., C. I. Fogel, and B. P. Black. 2013. "Comfort Levels of Active Duty Gay/Bisexual Male Service Members in the Military Healthcare System." *Military Medicine* 178(12): 1335–1340.

Birn, A-E., Y. Pillay, and T. H. Holtz. 2009. *Textbook of International Health: Global Health in a Dynamic World* (5th ed.). New York: Oxford University Press.

Black, S. A., M. S. Gallaway, and E. C. Ritchie. 2011. "Prevalence and Risk Factors Associated with Suicides of Army Soldiers 2001–2009." *Military Psychology* 23(4): 433–451.

Bliese, P. D., K. M. Wright, A. B. Adler, J. L. Thomas, and C. W. Hoge. 2007. "Timing of Postcombat Mental Health Assessments." *Psychological Services* 4(3): 141–148.

Blumenthal, S. 2012, September 14, updated 2017, December 6. "Stopping the Surge of Military Suicides: How to Win This Preventable War" [web log comment]. *Huffington Post*. Retrieved from www.huffingtonpost.com.

Booth, B., M. W. Segal, and D. B. Bell. 2007. *What We Know About Army Families: 2007 Update*. Washington, DC: Caliber and US Army.

Brown, G. R., and K. T. Jones. 2015. "Mental Health and Medical Health Disparities in 5135 Transgender Veterans Receiving Healthcare in the Veterans Health Administration: A Case-control Study." *LGBT Health* (December 16). doi:10.1089/lgbt.2015.0058.

Burks, D. J. 2011. "Lesbian, Gay, and Bisexual Victimization in the Military: An Unintended Consequence of 'Don't Ask, Don't Tell'?" *American Psychologist* 66(7): 604–613.

Burland, D., and J. H. Lundquist. 2013. "The Best Years of Our Lives: Military Service and Family Relationships—A Life Course Perspective." In J. M. Wilmoth and A. London (Eds.), *Life-Course Perspectives on Military Service* (pp. 1–37). New York and London: Routledge.

Centers for Disease Control and Prevention (CDC). 2015. "Leading Causes of Death (LCOD) by Age Group, All Males—United States, 2015." Retrieved from https://www.cdc.gov.

Chandra, A., S. Lara-Cinisomo, L. H. Jaycox, T. Tanielian, R. M. Burns, T. Ruder, and B. Han. 2009. "Children on the Homefront: The Experience of Children from Military Families." *Pediatrics* 125: 16–25.

Chartrand, M. M., D. A. Frank, L. F. White, and T. R. Shope. 2008. "Effect of Parents' Wartime Deployment on the Behavior of Young Children in Military Families." *Archives of Pediatrics and Adolescent Medicine* 162 (11): 1009–1014.

Cozza, S. J., J. M. Guimond, J.B.A. McKibben, R. S. Chan, Teresa L Aruta-Maiers, . . . R. J. Ursano. 2010. "Combat-injured Service Members and Their Families: The Relationship of Child Distress and Spouse-perceived Family Distress and Disruption." *Journal of Traumatic Stress* 23(1): 112–115.

CSAction. 2011, October 21. "CAB Landing Zones in Colorado." Retrieved from www.youtube.com.

Elbogen, E. B., H. R. Wagner, S. R. Fuller, P. S. Calhoun, P. M. Kinnear, Mid-Atlantic Mental Illness Research, Education, and Clinical Center Workgroup, and J. C. Beckham. 2010. "Correlates of Anger and Hostility in Iraq and Afghanistan War Veterans." *American Journal of Psychiatry* 167(9): 1051–1058.

Engel, R. C., L. B. Gallagher, and D. S. Lyle. 2010. "Military Deployments and Children's Academic Achievement: Evidence from Department of Defense Education Activity Schools." *Economics of Education Review* 29(1): 73–82.

Enloe, C. 2000. *Manuevers: The International Politics of Militarizing Women's Lives.* Berkeley: University of California Press.

Enloe, C. 2007. *Globalization and Militarism: Feminists Make the Link.* Lanham, MD: Rowan & Littlefield.

Enloe, C. 2010. *Nimo's War, Emma's War.* Berkeley: University of California Press.

Esposito-Smythers, C., J. Wolff, K. M. Lemmon, M. Bodzy, R. R. Swenson, and A. Spirito. 2011. "Military Youth and the Deployment Cycle: Emotional Health Consequences and Recommendations for Intervention." *Journal of Family Psychology* 25(4): 497–507.

Faber, A. J., E. Willerton, S. R. Clymer, S. M. MacDermid, and H. M. Weiss. 2008. "Ambiguous Absence, Ambiguous Presence: A Qualitative Study of Military Reserve Families in Wartime." *Journal of Family Psychology* 22(2): 222–230.

Farmer, P. 1999. *Infections and Inequalities: The Modern Plagues.* Berkeley: University of California Press.

Farmer, P. 2005. *Pathologies of Power: Health, Human Rights, and the New War on the Poor.* Berkeley: University of California Press.

Farmer, P., B. Nizeye, S. Stulac, and S. Keshavjee. 2006. "Structural Violence and Clinical Medicine." *PLOS Medicine* 3(10): e449.

Finley, B. 2017, July 25. "Air Force Admits Firefighting Foam that Was Spilled on Base Contaminated Water and Soil." *Denver Post,* July 25. Retrieved from www.denverpost.com.

Finley, E. P. 2011. *Fields of Combat: Understanding PTSD among Veterans of Iraq and Afghanistan.* Ithaca, NY: Cornell University Press.

Flake, E. M., B. E. Davis, P. L. Johnson, and L. Middleton. 2009. "The Psychosocial Effects of Deployment on Military Children." *Journal of Developmental and Behavioral Pediatrics* 30(4): 271–278.

Forster, L. 2018. "Fort Carson Fire 100 Percent Contained, Army Says." *Gazette,* April 9. Retrieved from http://gazette.com.

Gassmann, J.N.N. 2010. *Patrolling the Homefront: The Emotional Labor of Army Wives Volunteering in Family Readiness Groups* (Doctoral dissertation). Retrieved from kuscholarworks.ku.edu.

Goldbach, J. T., and C. A. Carl Castro. 2016. "Lesbian, Gay, Bisexual, and Transgender (LGBT) Service Members: Life after 'Don't Ask, Don't Tell.'" *Current Psychiatry Reports 18:* 56. doi: 10.1007/s11920-016-0695-0.

González, R. 2010. *Militarizing Culture: Essays on the Warfare State.* Walnut Creek, CA: Left Coast Press.

Gorman, G. H., M. Eide, and E. Hisle-Gorman. 2010. "Wartime Military Deployment and Increased Pediatric Mental and Behavioral Health Complaints." *Pediatrics* 126(6): 1058–1066.

Gottman, J. M., J. S. Gottman, and C. L. Atkins. 2011. "The Comprehensive Soldier Fitness Program: Family Skills Component." *American Psychologist* 66(1): 52.

Gutmann, M. C., and C. Lutz. 2010. *Breaking Ranks: Iraq Veterans Speak Out Against the War.* Berkeley: University of California Press.

Hahn, R. A. 1999. "Anthropology and the Enhancement of Public Health Practice." In R. B. Hahn (Ed.), *Anthropology in Public Health: Bridging Differences in Culture and Society*, (pp. 3–26). New York and Oxford: Oxford University Press.

Hautzinger, S., and J. Scandlyn. 2014. *Beyond Post-Traumatic Stress: Homefront Struggles with the Wars on Terror*. Walnut Creek, CA: Left Coast Press.

Huebner, A. J., and J. A. Mancini. 2005. "Adjustments among Adolescents in Military Families When a Parent Is Deployed: A Final Report Submitted to the Military Family Research Institute and Department of Defense Quality of Life Office." Falls Church: Virginia Tech, Department of Human Development.

Huebner, A. J., J. A. Mancini, R. M. Wilcox, S. R. Grass, and G. A. Grass. 2007. "Parental Deployment and Youth in Military Families: Exploring Uncertainty and Ambiguous Loss." *Family Relations* 56(2): 112–122.

Hynes, H. P. 2011. "Military Hazardous Waste Sickens Land and People." *Truthout*, August 4. Retrieved from www.truth-out.org.

Katz, K. A. 2010. "Health Hazards of 'Don't Ask, Don't Tell.'" *New England Journal of Medicine* 363: 2380–2381.

Keller, C. A. 2006. "Prologue: Legacies." In A. Crossley and C. A. Keller, *The Army Wife Handbook* (pp. xx–xxxi). Marietta, GA: ABI Press.

Killgore, W D.S., D. I. Cotting, J. L. Thomas, A. L. Cox, D. McGurk, A. H. Vo, . . . C. W. Hoge. 2008. "Post-Combat Invincibility: Violent Combat Experiences Are Associated with Increased Risk-taking Propensity following Deployment." *Journal of Psychiatric Research* 42(13): 1112–1121.

Knobloch, L. K., K. B. Pusateri, A. T. Ebata, and P. C. McGlaughlin. 2015. "Experiences of Military Youth during a Family Member's Deployment: Changes, Challenges, and Opportunities." *Youth and Society* 47(3): 319–342.

Krieger, N. 1994. "Epidemiology and the Web of Causation: Has Anyone Seen the Spider?" *Social Science and Medicine* 39(7): 887–903.

Kriner, D. L., and F. X. Shen. 2010. *The Casualty Gap: The Causes and Consequences of American Wartime Inequalities*. New York: Oxford University Press.

Lester, P., P. J. Reeves, L. Knauss, D. Glover, and C. Mogil. 2010. "The Long War and Parental Combat Deployment: Effects on Military Children and At-home Spouses." *Journal of the American Academy of Child and Adolescent Psychiatry* 49: 310–320.

Litz, B. T., N. Stein, E. Delaney, L. Lebowitz, W. P. Nash, C. Silva, and S. Maguen. 2009. "Moral Injury and Moral Repair in War Veterans: A Preliminary Model and Intervention Strategy." *Clinical Psychology Review* 29(8): 695–706.

Lusk, J., L. A. Brenner, L. M. Betthauser, H. Terrio, A. I. Scher, K. A. Schwab, and A. Poczwardowski. 2015. "A Qualitative Study of Potential Suicide Risk Factors among Operation Iraqi Freedom/Operation Enduring Freedom Soldiers Returning to the Continental United States (CONUS)." *Journal of Clinical Psychology* 71(9): 843–855.

Lutz, C., and K. Millar. 2012. War. In D. Fassin (Ed.), *A Companion to Moral Anthropology* (pp. 482–499). Oxford: Wiley-Blackwell.

MacLeish, K. T. 2013. *Making War at Fort Hood: Life and Uncertainty in a Military Community*. Princeton, NJ: Princeton University Press.

Maguen, S., and B. Litz. 2012. "Moral Injury in Veterans of War." *PTSD Research Quarterly* 23(1): 1–3.
Mansfield, A. J., J. S. Kaufman, S. W. Marshall, B. N. Gaynes, J. P. Morrissey, and C. C. Engel. 2010. "Deployment and the Use of Mental Health Services among U.S. Army Wives." *New England Journal of Medicine* 362(2): 101–109.
Marshall, A. D., J. Panuzio, and C. T. Taft. 2005. "Intimate Partner Violence among Military Veterans and Active Duty Servicemen." *Clinical Psychology Review* 25(7): 862–876.
Mash, H. B., C. S. Haberman, H. Fullerton, J. Ramsawh, T.H.H. Ng, L. Wang, . . . R. J. Ursano. 2014. "Risk for Suicidal Behaviors Associated with Alcohol and Energy Drink Use in the US Army." *Social Psychiatry and Psychiatric Epidemiology* 49(9): 1379–1387.
Moore, C. 2015, April 25. "Fort Carson Solider [sic] Killed in Colorado Springs Motorcycle, Truck Collision." *KDVR Fox 31*. Retrieved from kdvr.com.
Naclerio, A. L. 2015. "Medical Issues for Women Warriors on Deployment." In E. C. Ritchie and A. L. Naclerio (Eds.), *Women at War* (pp. 49–77). Oxford: Oxford University Press.
National Military Family Association (NMFA). 2008. "10 Things Military Teens Want You to Know." Retrieved from support.militaryfamily.org.
Negrusa, S., B. Negrusa, and J. Hosek. 2014. "Gone to War: Have Deployments Increased Divorces?" *Journal of Population Economics* 27: 473–496.
Ostrach, B. and M. Singer 2013. "Syndemics of War: Malnutrition-Infectious Disease Interactions and the Unintended Health Consequences of Intentional Health Policies." *Annals of Anthropological Practice* 36(2): 257–273. American Anthropological Association. doi:10.1111/napa.12003.
Ramchand, R., J. Miles, T. Schell, L. Jaycox, G.N. Marshall, and T. Tanielian. 2011. "Prevalence and Correlates of Drinking Behaviors of Previously Deployed Military Personnel and Matched Civilian Population." *Military Psychology* 23(1): 6–21.
Reuben, S. H. 2010. *Reducing Environmental Cancer Risk*. U.S. Department of Health and Human Service, National Institutes of Health, National Cancer Institute. Retrieved from deainfo.nci.nih.gov.
Ruckart, P. Z., F. J. Bove, and M. Maslia. 2013. "Evaluation of Exposure to Contaminated Drinking Water and Specific Birth Defects and Childhood Cancers at Marine Corps Base Camp Lejeune, North Carolina: A Case-control Study." *Environmental Health* 12: 104. Retrieved from ehjournal.biomedcentral.com.
Scarry, E. 1985. *The Body in Pain: The Making and Unmaking of the World*. Oxford: Oxford University Press.
Sciencecorps. 2012. "Health Hazards of Chemicals Commonly Used on Military Bases." Retrieved from www.sciencecorps.org.
Scott, J. 2010. "Mothers in the Military: Punishing Mothers Who Serve" (Web log comment). *POV: Regarding War Blog*, April 13. Retrieved from www.pbs.org.
Sherman, M., and U. Bowling. 2011. "Challenges and Opportunities for Intervening with Couples in the Aftermath of the Global War on Terrorism." *Journal of Contemporary Psychotherapy* 41(4): 209–217.

Thorpe, H. 2014. *Soldier Girls: The Battles of Three Women at Home and at War.* New York: Scribner.
Tolkien, J.R.R. 1997 [1937]. *The Hobbit or Here and Back Again.* New York: Houghton Mifflin.
TriWest Group. 2011. *The Status of Behavioral Health Care in Colorado—2011 Update.* Denver: Advancing Colorado's Mental Health Care: Caring for Colorado Foundation, The Colorado Health Foundation, The Colorado Trust, and The Denver Foundation.
US Army War College (USAWC). 2009. *Battle Book IV: A Guide for Spouses in Leadership Roles.* Retrieved from www.armywarcollege.edu.
Vatic Project. 2011. "Stop the Pentagon's 51st State." September 27. Retrieved from vaticproject.blogspot.com.
Waterston, A. 2009. "On War and Accountability." In A. Waterston (Ed.), *An Anthropology of War: Views from War Zones* (pp. 12–31). New York: Berghahn Books.
Weinstein, L., and C. White. 1997. *Wives and Warriors: Women and the Military in the United States and Canada.* Westport, CT: Bergin and Garvey.
Wilk, J. E., P. D. Bliese, P. Y. Kim, J. L. Thomas, D. McGurk, and C. W. Hoge. 2010. "Relationship of Combat Experiences to Alcohol Misuse among US Soldiers Returning from the Iraq War." *Drug and Alcohol Dependence* 108(1): 115–121.
Wool, Z. H. 2015. *After War: The Weight of Life at Walter Reed.* Durham, NC: Duke University Press.
World Health Organization (WHO). 1948. *Preamble to the Constitution of the World Health Organization.* As adopted by the International Health Conference, New York, June 19–22, 1946, and entered into force on April 7, 1948.

APPENDIX

The Body Count

NETA CRAWFORD

TABLE A.1. Direct Deaths in Major War Zones: Afghanistan and Pakistan (October 2001–October 2018) and Iraq (March 2003–October 2018)[1]

	Afghanistan	Pakistan	Iraq	Total
US Military[2]	2,401[3]		4,550[4]	6,951
US DOD Civilian Casualties[5]	6		15	21
US Contractors[6]	3,937	90	3,793	7,820
National Military and Police[7]	58,596[8]	8,832[9]	41,726[10]	109,154
Other Allied Troops[11]	1,141		323	1,464
Civilians	38,480[12]	23,372[13]	182,272–204,575[14]	244,124–266,427
Opposition Fighters	42,100[15]	32,490[16]	34,806–39,881[17]	109,396–114,471
Journalists/Media Workers[18]	54	63	245[19]	362
Humanitarian/ NGO Workers[20]	409	95	62[21]	566
TOTAL	147,124	64,942	267,792–295,170	479,858–507,236
TOTAL (rounded to nearest 1,000)	147,000	65,000	268,000–295,000[22]	480,000–507,000

1 This chart tallies direct deaths, caused by war violence. It does not include indirect deaths, namely those caused by loss of access to food, water, and/or infrastructure, war-related disease, etc. The numbers included here are approximations based on the reporting of several original data sources. Not all data sources are updated through mid-October 2018; dates are noted in the footnotes. These footnotes document the ways in which some original data sources are incomplete, inconsistent, and/or where data are inaccessible. For example, it is impossible to separate numbers of US military service members who died in Iraq from those who died in Syria, as the Department of Defense includes those in the same category. For this reason, this chart includes US service members who have died in Syria but does not include others who have died in Syria due to the US-led war on terror, such as Syrian civilians.

2 Department of Defense. 2018. Department of Defense Casualty Report. Retrieved from https://dod.defense.gov/ (data through October 19, 2018) in Afghanistan (Operations Enduring Freedom and Freedom's Sentinel) and Iraq (Operations Iraqi Freedom, New Dawn, and Inherent Resolve).

3 Figures for US military deaths in Afghanistan operations include 131 deaths in other operational locations, including Pakistan.

4 Figures for US military deaths in Iraq Operations after August 2014 (in Operation Inherent Resolve) include deaths in other operational locations, including Syria.

5 US Department of Defense. 2018. Department of Defense Casualty Report. Retrieved from https://dod.defense.gov/news (data through October 19, 2018). Figures include deaths in other operational locations.

6 US Department of Labor (DOL). 2018. Defense Base Act Case Summary by Nation. Retrieved from www.dol.gov (data through September 30, 2018). DOL data for contractor deaths in Iraq are 1,664; in Afghanistan, 1,734; and for Pakistan 42. These DOL figures do not include other DOL-reported deaths likely connected to the named military operations in Iraq and Afghanistan, including contractor deaths in Kuwait (103), Jordan (36), Qatar (19), Saudi Arabia (23), Syria (5), United Arab Emirates (13) and elsewhere which are included in the present estimate. The figures here are an estimate of contractor deaths based on these DOL numbers which calculates the additional number of unreported contractor deaths by comparing the percentage of foreign contractors working for the US military in the war zone with the much lower percentage of foreign contractors among the reported dead. The multiplier reflecting this disparity is 2.15 times the DOL number.

7 Includes National Military Forces and National and Local Police Forces.

8 There is uncertainty about the number of Afghan National Police and military deaths. This estimate is based on several sources, including the Brookings Institution, "Afghanistan Index"; *New York Times*; and US Government, Special Inspector General Reports on Afghanistan. The *New York Times* reported 13,729 Afghan National Security and Police deaths from 2001 to 2014. See Rod Nordland, "War Deaths Top 13,000 in Afghan Security Forces," *New York Times*, March 3, 2014. For trends, see I. S. Livingston and M. O'Hanlon, 2017. Afghanistan Index, fig. 1.15, p. 12. Retrieved from www.brookings.edu. With the US drawdown since 2014, Afghan military, police, and other security forces have borne an increasing share of the combat and are now more exposed to militant attacks. See Neta C. Crawford, 2015, "War Related Death, Injury and Displacement in Afghanistan and Pakistan 2001–2014." *Costs of War* website. Retrieved from https://watson.brown.edu. In January 2017, the Special Inspector General for Afghanistan Reconstruction (SIGAR) reported 6,785 Afghan National Defense and Security Forces (ANDSF) killed from January 1, 2016 to November 12, 2016: www.sigar.mil. US forces in Afghanistan began to classify these numbers in 2017 after previously releasing them. See Thomas Gibbons-Neff, "Afghan War Data, Once Public, Is Censored in U.S. Military Report," *New York Times*, October 30, 2017; Rod Nordland, "The Death Toll for Afghan Forces Is Secret. Here's Why," *New York Times*, September 21, 2018. In December 2017, the DOD reported that the "number of ANDSF casualties suffered while conducting local patrols and checkpoint operations was similar to that of 2016," while "the number of casualties in planned operations has decreased over the same period." Department of Defense, Enhancing Security and Stability in Afghanistan: www.defense.gov. See Special Inspector General for Afghanistan Reconstruction (SIGAR), SIGAR Quarterly Report, April 30, 2018. Retrieved from www.sigar.mil.

9 Through 2017 from Pak Institute for Peace Studies (PIPS). 2017. Pak Institute for Peace Studies Annual *Pakistan Security Reports*. Retrieved from http://pakpips.com.

10 Most sources consider their numbers an undercount of the actual total. This estimate includes 8,825 deaths recorded by iCasualties, for January 2005 to July 2011, and 1,300 deaths prior to 2005. Agence France Presse gives a total from August 2011 to January 2015 of 5,601 army and policy deaths, using Iraqi government figures. See https://docs.google.com. However, the government numbers are assessed by Iraq Body Count to be a significant undercount. Moreover, this is an amorphous category—some local militias work with the Iraqi police and military. Leith Aboufadel, "Over 26,000 Iraqi Soldiers Killed in 4 Year War with ISIS," *Almasdar News*, December 13, 2017. Retrieved from https://docs.google.com.

11 iCasualties (data through 2018, October 19). Retrieved from http://icasualties.org.

12 For 2003–2007, see Crawford, "War Related Death, Injury and Displacement in Afghanistan and Pakistan 2001–2014"; for 2008–2017, see the United Nations Assistance Mission in Afghanistan (UNAMA) annual *Reports on the Protection of Civilians in Armed Conflict*, retrieved from https://unama.unmissions.org. These civilian death numbers include the recorded direct violent deaths. Additional direct violent deaths may not have been recorded and significant numbers of indirect deaths due to displacement or destruction of infrastructure have not been included.

13 Pak Institute for Peace Studies (PIPS), 2017. Pak Institute for Peace Studies Annual *Pakistan Security Reports*. Retrieved from http://pakpips.com. These data are mostly consistent with South Asia Terrorism Portal, 2018, "Fatalities in Terrorist Violence in Pakistan 2003–2018." Retrieved from www.satp.org. The counts of the

dead (and wounded) are complicated not only by the difficulty of access to war zones for investigators, but also because some actors have incentives either to exaggerate or to minimize the number of civilians killed, or to identify civilians as militants.

14 This is surely an underestimate of the direct deaths in the wars in Iraq and does not include the number of civilians killed in Syria. We use the most conservative numbers, produced by Iraq Body Count tally through September 2018. Retrieved from www.iraqbodycount.org. IBC has verified their count through January 2017 and says that a complete analysis of Wikileaks data may add as many as 10,000 deaths. In August 2018, the United States acknowledged that it killed at least 1,114 civilians in the fight against ISIS in Iraq and Syria since their intervention there in August 2014. Borzou Daragahi, "Pentagon Admits War on Isis Has Killed More Than 1,100 Civilians in Syria and Iraq." *Independent*, September 27, 2018. Retrieved from www.independent.co.uk. Worse, there are potentially thousands of bodies buried in rubble from bombardment in Iraq whose deaths may never be recorded. See Patrick Cockburn, "The Massacre of Mosul: 40,000 Feared Dead in Battle to Take Back City from ISIS as Scale of Civilian Casualties Revealed," *Independent*, July 19, 2017. Retrieved from www.independent.co.uk. Some of the most consistent reporting of casualties caused by Coalition and Russian air strikes is at the Airwars website at https://airwars.

15 An estimate calculated from 185 Afghanistan Ministry of Defense press releases from January 1, 2015 to December 31, retrieved from http://mod.gov.af. Neither the United States or NATO have released figures on the exact number of anti-government insurgents killed. See also Crawford, "War Related Death, Injury and Displacement in Afghanistan and Pakistan."

16 Through 2017. See Pak Institute for Peace Studies (PIPS). 2017. Pak Institute for Peace Studies (PIPS) annual *Pakistan Security Reports*. Retrieved from http://pakpips.com.

17 Estimating that about 9,200 Iraqi soldiers (plus or minus 1,600) were killed in 2003 resisting the US invasion and initial occupation, and that about 19,000 militants were killed from 2003 to September 2007. Iraq Body Count found 20,499 "enemy" deaths in Iraq War Logs, from January 2004 through December 2009. See Carl Conetta, "The Wages of War: Iraqi Combatant and Noncombatant Fatalities in the 2003 Conflict." Project on Defense Alternatives Research Monograph, #8, October 20, 2003. Retrieved from https://reliefweb.int; and Jim Michaels, "Thousands of Enemy Fighters Reported Killed," *USA TODAY*, September 27, 2007. Retrieved from www.usatoday.com; Iraq Body Count, "Iraq War Log Analysis: What the Numbers Reveal," October 23, 2010. Retrieved from www.iraqbodycount.org. Agence France Press cites Iraqi sources as saying 14,239 militants were killed from January 2006 through January 2015; https://docs.google.com. I add an estimated average of 500–1,000 militants killed each year from January 2015 to October 2018.

18 Journalist and media worker deaths for war years through September 2018. See Committee to Protect Journalists (CPJ) (2018). Retrieved from https://cpj.org/data (Journalist Motive Confirmed and Media Workers Motive Confirmed and Unconfirmed).

19 Since 2024, 62 journalists and media workers have been killed in Syria.

20 The Aid Worker Security Database (Last updated August 9, 2018,). National and International Aid Workers Killed. Retrieved from https://aidworkersecurity.org.

21 This total does not include the 138 aid workers who have been killed in Syria since August 1, 2014.

22 The total does not include the more than 500,000 people estimated killed in the civil war in Syria from March 2011 through March 2018. More than 110,000 of these were civilians; see Syrian Observatory for Human Rights, 2018, "About 522 Thousand People Were Killed in 90 Months Since the Start of the Syrian Revolution in March 1990." Retrieved from www.syriahr.com. See also Agence France Press. "Syria War Has Killed More than 350,000 in 7 Years: Monitor," *Daily Mail*, March 12, 2018. Retrieved from www.dailymail.co.uk.

ABOUT THE EDITORS

CATHERINE LUTZ is Thomas J. Watson Jr. Family Professor of Anthropology and International Studies at Brown University, and writes on security and militarization, gender violence, and transportation. She is Co-director of the Costs of War Project, a collaborative assessment of wars' consequences. She has consulted with civil society organizations as well as with the UN Department of Peacekeeping Operations and the government of Guam and is a former Guggenheim Fellow and Radcliffe Fellow.

ANDREA MAZZARINO is a social worker and human rights activist with interests in the health impacts of war and in children's and disability rights. She has held various clinical and research positions, including as co-founder of Brown University's Costs of War Project, as a clinician at the Veterans Affairs PTSD Outpatient Clinic, and as a researcher and independent consultant with Human Rights Watch's Europe & Central Asia Division.

ABOUT THE CONTRIBUTORS

Ghassan Soleiman Abu-Sittah, MD, is Assistant Professor of Clinical Surgery, Plastic Surgery at the American University of Beirut Medical Center, and he is Co-Director of the Conflict Medicine Program at the Global Health Institute.

Svea Closser is Associate Professor at Middlebury College, and a medical anthropologist whose research focuses on the interaction between global health policy and local health systems.

Noah Coburn is Associate Professor at Bennington College, and a sociocultural anthropologist focusing on Afghanistan as well as political structures and violence in the Middle East and Central Asia.

Neta Crawford is Professor of Political Science at Boston University and Co-Director of the Costs of War Project. Her research focuses on the fate of civilians in war, international ethics, and normative change.

Anila Daulatzai is a sociocultural anthropologist with extensive research experience in both Afghanistan and Pakistan, with a focus on war, humanitarianism, gender, violence, and care.

Scott Harding is Associate Professor at the University of Connecticut School of Social Work and a specialist on war, militarism, forced migration, and social work.

Sarah Hautzinger is Professor at Colorado College and an ethnographer and political anthropologist whose research is concerned with power, difference, and in/equality, particularly gender and violence.

About the Contributors

MARCIA C. INHORN is the William K. Lanman, Jr. Professor of Anthropology and International Affairs at Yale University, specializing in Middle Eastern gender, religion, and health.

KATHRYN LIBAL is Associate Professor of Social Work and Human Rights at the University of Connecticut and Director of the Human Rights Institute, specializing in human rights, humanitarianism and migration, and social welfare in the Middle East and United States.

KYLEA LAINA LIESE is a medical anthropologist and certified nurse midwife at the University of Illinois, Chicago, focused on the social drivers and repercussions of maternal morbidity and mortality.

KEN MACLEISH is an anthropologist and Assistant Professor at Vanderbilt University focused on soldier and veteran health.

LAYTH MULA-HUSSAIN is a radiation oncologist at the Cross Cancer Institute and the Slemani Radiation Oncology Center in Iraq.

PATRICIA OMIDIAN has worked as an applied medical anthropologist in Afghanistan and Pakistan since 1997. She has served as Children and War Advisor for Save the Children United States.

CATHERINE PANTER-BRICK is Professor of Anthropology, Health, and Global Affairs at Yale University. She is a medical anthropologist who has published extensively on trauma and mental health in Afghanistan and has performed other extensive global health research.

JEAN SCANDLYN is Research Associate Professor in the Departments of Health and Behavioral Sciences and Anthropology at the University of Colorado, Denver and a medical anthropologist focused on global health, migration, and healthcare.

MAC SKELTON is a medical anthropologist and Director of Research and Policy at the Institute of Regional and International Studies at the

American University of Iraq, Sulaimani. His work has focused on cancer and its social and wartime contexts of care.

ZOË H. WOOL is Assistant Professor of Anthropology at Rice University whose research focuses on the experiences of injured American soldiers and veterans and their family members as well as on care and disability more broadly.

INDEX

Afghanistan, 1, 3–5, 14, 16, 19–22, 26–30, 41–107: Afghan Ministry of Martyrs and Social Welfare, 73; aid worker violence, 90–106; American veterans, 14; Badakhshan, 44–49, 53; "brain drain," 54n3; British Empire, 59; childbirth, 41–54; civilian medical NGOs, 22; civil war, 45, 50; Deash, 68, 160; Democratic Republic of Afghanistan, 44; drone strikes, 26, 58–70; fatwa, 65–66; *Focusing*, 94, 102–3, 105; healthcare, 3, 21, 27, 62; health worker attacks, 67–68, 90–91; heroin economy, 73–85; humanitarian aid, 90–106; infrastructure, 5, 11, 19; internally displaced persons, 27; Islamic State of Afghanistan, 44; Kabul, 73, 77–85; Kabul University, 79; marriage age, 50–51; maternal mortality, 41; mental health, 9; mujahideen, 48–50; occupation by the Soviet Union, 43, 45, 59, 62, 76, 92; polio, 57–58, 63–70; Shari'a law, 48; Soviet invasion, 3; status of women, 41–54; substance abuse, 8; suicide, 8; Taliban, 42–46, 48–49, 61, 67–68, 76; US invasion, 3; US-led occupation, 26, 79. vaccines, 68–69; war in Iraq, Afghanistan, and Pakistan, 1, 4, 16, 22, 27–29; war with Soviet Union, 43; widows, 73–85. *See also* serial war
Air Force, 245
All-Volunteer Force (AVF), 244
Al-Hashd militia, 146
Al Maliki, Nouri, 158
al Qaeda, in Iraq, 115, 141
al-Sadr, Moqtada, 115
al-Sistani, Ayatollah, Al-Hashd militia of, 146
Althusser, Louis, 147
American University of Beirut Medical Center (AUBMC), 137, 143–48, 161–68

Battle Deaths Dataset, 139
BearingPoint Inc. (formerly KPMG Consulting), 127
Bechtel, 127
bin Laden, Osama, 7, 65
Black feminist thought, 216
"brain drain": in Afghanistan, 45, 54n3; in Iraq, 25, 114, 123–24
Bremer, Paul, 126–27
Brookings Institution, 60
Brown University, 140
Bureau of Investigative Journalism, 60
Bush administration, 58, 116, 127

cancer care in Iraq, 152–68, 172–85: bone marrow transplants, 153, 158, 162–65; depleted uranium (DU), 154, 174, 181; drug shortage, 174; exodus of doctors, 156; financial resources, 183; government sponsorship, 167; Hiwa Cancer Hospital, 157, 164; Nanakali Cancer Hospital, 157, 164; reconstructive surgeries, 153; top ten cancers, 176–81
CARE International, 79–82, 128
Castro, Carl, 202
"casualty gap," 244

265

266 | INDEX

Center for Environmental Health Studies, 180–81
Centers for Disease Control, 198
chemical weapons, 22–23, 26: cancer treatments, 156, 175; environmental pollution, 23, 26; human health outcomes, 15, 26; "radiogenic communities," 14
children: Angolan civil war, 19, 30; mortality, 173; parent deployment, 234–35; wartime domestic violence, 18
civilians, 1, 232: casualties, 255–57; casualties in Iraq, 116, 141; drone casualties, 58–59; guilt, 193–94; reintegration, 239–40; suicide rate, 191
colonialism, in South Asia, Africa, and the Middle East, 43
Colorado Springs, 232–49: domestic violence, 242; Rocky Mountain Arsenal, 245; Veterans Trauma Court, 243
combatants, 1, 156; casualties, 255–57
Conflict Medicine Program, 138
contractors, 192
Correlates of War Project, 139
Costs of War Project, 2–3, n71, 140

Daesh, 68, 160
death, conflict-related, 1, 3, 5–7, 255–57
"de-Baathification," 126
Department of Defense, 245
disability care collective, 215
domestic violence: in Afghanistan, 18; in the military, 231, 242, 243; among Syrian refugees in Iraq, 122
Don't Ask Don't Tell, 214, 233, 247–48
drone strikes, 57–70; in Afghanistan and Pakistan, 26, 57–70; Central Intelligence Agency (CIA), 60; civilian casualties, 58–60; signature strikes, 60
drug use, 74–85; addiction trajectories, 77; dependency, 79; heroin, 74–85; War on Drugs, 76, 82

ecological impact, 244: Superfund sites, 244
education, 13
environment: base-building, 15; hazards of warfare, 180; waste, 15–16, 23
Esfandiari, Mohammad, 139

family life, military, 214–19: male spouses, 237; marriage and divorce, 238–39; military family, 218–19; spouses' health, 236; wives' clubs, 237
fatwa: on polio, 65–66; on women, 91
financial distress, 240
First Gulf War, 24, 113, 118, 172, 181
Fort Carson, 231, 242; injury prevention program, 242; LGBTQ soldiers, 233–34
Fort Hood, 200
Foucault, Michel, 147, 192

Gates Foundation, 64
Geneva Declaration on Armed Violence and Development, 1
Germany, 178
Great Britain, combat in Iraq, 141
Guatemala, 43

Handicap International, 141
healthcare: in Afghanistan and Pakistan, 41, 62, 70; cancer patients, 11; kin and social networks, 18, 42, 47, 84, 154, 166–67; military healthcare in the United States, 3; obstetric, 44, 46; physical disabilities, 128; political capital, 138, 144, 146; reproductive, 42; social welfare state, 140; "therapeutic geography," 154; violence against workers, 123
heroin economy, 73–85
HIV/AIDS, 10–11, 216, 232
Hoge, Charles, 202
homicide rates, 243
humanitarian assistance: dilemmas, 93–94, 97–99; *Focusing*, 94, 102–3, 105; in healthcare, 21, 28; in Liberia, 21; in

Pakistan, 90–106; training workshops, 94, 99–103; violence against workers, 90–92, 104; in violent conflict, 25

Hussein, Saddam, 113–14, 126, 148; "Saddam's *Qaddisiyah*," 139; "Saddam's war of aggression," 139

Improvised Explosive Devises (IEDs), 210, 231: in Afghanistan, 30

India, 142, 153, 158, 166; Iraqis in, 158; Martyrs Fund, 142; New Delhi, 157

Indonesia, 44

infant mortality, 173

Inhorn, Marcia, 111, 129

Injury Severity Scores (ISS), 149, 149n2

insurgents, 156

internally displaced persons (IDPs), 7, 13, 91–92, 94–97, 105, 122; in Afghanistan, 27

International Committee of the Red Cross (ICRC), 116, 120, 141

International Medical Corps, 128

International Tribune, 90

Iran-Iraq War (or Iraq-Iran War), 113, 118, 139–40, 144, 148

Iran's Martyrs and Disabled Veterans' Organization, 139

Iraq: 2003 US invasion, 112, 114–16, 126, 129, 131, 137, 139, 165, 167, 172, 175; Abadi government, 143, 146; American veterans, 14; al-Askari Mosque, 141; "Awakening Councils," 115; Baghdad, 121, 157, 173; "Baghdad Security Plan," 114; civilian casualties and deaths, 116, 255–57; civil war, 141, 145; Coalition Provisional Authority, 126; the Compensation Law, 142; disability crisis, 128–29; ethnic cleansing, 113; Federal Police Force, 142; First Gulf War, 24, 113, 118, 172, 181; food insecurity, 120; government, 12–13; Hashd Shaabi (Popular Mobilization Forces), 161; health infrastructure, 12, 19, 25, 112–13, 118–20, 123, 130; infant mortality, 121; Iran-Iraq War (or Iraq-Iran War), 113, 118, 139–40, 144, 148; Iraqi Doctors' Syndicate, 123; Jihad Service Law, 140; Kirkuk, 116; life expectancy, 118; Maliki government, 143, 145; "martyrs," 139–40, 142; Martyrs Foundation, 143, 146; medical migration, 123–25, 137; mental health, 122; Ministry of Defense, 139; Ministry of Education, 121; Ministry of Health (IMOH), 12, 125, 137, 142–46, 152, 158, 173, 181, 184; Ministry of Higher Education and Scientific Research, 184; Ministry of Interior, 142–43, 145, 148; mobile clinics, 114; privatization, 127; religious minority groups, 114; "Report of the Iraq Inquiry," UK commissioned, 130; roles of NGOs, 124–129; "sectarianization," 113; Shi'a, 113–15, 125, 141; Sunni, 113–14, 125, 141, 144, 161; US trade embargo, 113; war and health, 111–131; waterborne diseases, 120, Yazidi, 130

Iraq Body Count (IBC), 117, 140–41

Iraq Family Health Survey Study Group, 149n1

Iraqi Cancer Board (ICB), 182–84

Iraqi Cancer Registry (ICR), 175–81

Iraqi Ministry of Health (IMOH), 12, 125, 137, 142–46, 152, 158, 173, 181, 184

Iraqi National Cancer Control Program five-year plan (INCCP for 2010–2014), 182–84

Iraqi Royal Medical College, 173

Islamic Republic of Iran, 139, 143, 153, 178; Tehran, 157

Islamic State of Iraq and the Levant (ISIL), 172–73; takeover of Mosul, 145

Islamic State of Iraq and Syria (ISIS), 130–31, 143–46, 161

Japan, 178

Johns Hopkins University, 117

Jordan, 114, 122, 153–54, 158, 178; Iraqis in, 158; Martyrs Fund, 142

Khomeini, Ruhollah, 148
kin and social networks, 18, 42, 47, 84, 154, 166–67
Kurds, 131–32n2, 153: Kurdish Regional Government (KRG), 157, 160
Kuwait, 124, 178

The Lancet, 117n149
Lebanon, 122, 152–53, 158; Beirut, 157–68; Iraqis in, 122, 152–53, 157–68; Martyrs Fund, 142; oncology in, 167
Libya, 137

"martyrs," 139–40, 142
maternal mortality, 7, 9; in Afghanistan, 27–28, 41–44, 51; internally displaced persons, 27–28; obstetric care, 18; in wartime, 11
MedAct, 124
Medecins Sans Frontieres, 114
"medical tourism," 153–54
mental illness, 9; children, 121; in Iraq, 121; military personnel and veterans, 211, 233, 239–43; military suicide, 192–96; posttraumatic stress disorder (PTSD), 9, 239–43, 247; services for refugees, 122; substance abuse, 75; US-led war in Iraq, 26
Mercy Corps, 128
military biopolitics, 191–205
"military-civilian gap," 244
military suicide, 191–205, 220–26; Army Public Health Service card, 200–201; care, 221–26; notion of risk, 200; policymakers, 191; US Active Duty Military Service Member Suicide Event Reports 2011–2017, 197*f*; US Army's 2010 suicide prevention report, 193
Moynihan Report, 216
Murcos, Shawqi Sabri, 155

narrative of the war-wounded, 146–47: American sub-stratification, 149; war wound as form or *bio-interpellation*, 147, Soviet, 149
National Cancer Act of 1971, 184–85
National Intelligence Estimate, 142
neoliberalism, 83; and economic development, 232; reconstruction policies, 113, 126–29; "regime of resilience," 84
New America Foundation, 60
New England Journal of Medicine, n149
New York City, 1

Obama administration, 58, 60
Outward Bound, 249n3

Pakistan, 1–4, 6, 8; drones, 26, 57–61; Federally Administered Tribal Areas (FATA), 59, 92, 94–5; Hafiz Gul Bahadar (cleric), 65–66; health, 22, 26–28; Kashmir, 59, 62, 93; Khyber Pakhtunkhwa (KPK), 59, 90, 92, 94; North Waziristan, 65; Peshawar, 95
Parsons Delaware Inc., 127
"patients without borders," 154
Phillips, David L., 126
Physicians for Social Responsibility, 131
Piñon Canyon Maneuver Site (PCMS), 245
polio, 57–70; in children, 68; Global Polio Eradication Initiative, 57, 62; health worker murders, 65; international funding for, 64; vaccinations, 57, 63–65; "War on Polio," 76, 86n2
political economy, 111
posttraumatic stress disorder (PTSD), 8; children, 121; and depression, 239–43, 247; military suicide, 197, 222; veterans, 210–12, 231–33, 240

Quran, 80, 103

rape, 1, 10, 13; in the military, 248
Reagan, Ronald, 148

refugees: Afghans, 27, 92; domestic violence, 122; internally displaced persons (IDPs), 7, 13, 91–92, 94–97, 105, 122; Iraqis, 114, 122; Jalozai camp, 96, 105; mental illness, 103, 122; movement to Europe, 168; in Pakistan, 92; PTSD in, 8; and rape, 10; in Syria, 122. *See also* United Nations High Commissioner for Refugees

Rotary International, 64

Saddam Center for the Diagnosis, Treatment, and Research of Tumors, 181
Second Battalion, Seventh Marine Regiment, 225
September 11, 2001, 1
serial war, 73–78, 81–82, 83–84
Shi'a, 113–15, 125, 141
Society for Medical Anthropology, 111
Sogn, Emily, 198
Soviet Union, 148; Great Patriotic War, 149
Special Inspector General for Iraq Reconstruction (SIGIR), 127
Sufism, 102
suicide bombing, 141
suicide rate, 195–205
Sunni, 113–14, 125, 141, 144, 161
Syria, 114, 122, 130
"syndemics of war," 5–6, 129–30, 249

Taliban: in Afghanistan, 42–46, 48–49, 61, 67–68, 76; insurgency, 92; in Pakistan, 59, 65–66, 91–95, 98
"terrorism," 142, 144
TriCARE (military health insurance), 241
Turkey, 143, 153, 158; Iraqis in, 158; Istanbul, 157

United Nations, 116, 119–22: sanctions in Iraq, 155–56, 172, 174; UNICEF, 46, 57, 90, 119; UNICEF Special Representative for Iraq, 119–20; UN Women, 93
United Nations High Commissioner for Refugees (UNHCR), 7, 96
US Agency for International Development (USAID), 127
US National Counterterrorism Center, 141

veterans: chronic pain, 211–13; with disabilities, 139, 210–26; female caregivers, 217; female veterans, 215; high-risk activities, 241–42; Iraq and Afghanistan, 14; post-9/11, 210; reintegration, 240–49; suicide, 191–205, 220–26; VA, 212–26; wounded, 144, 146; Vietnam War, 203

Walter Reed Army Medical Center, 215
war memorials, 246
"war on terror," 57, 75, 156: in Afghanistan, Iraq, and Pakistan, 1, 3
Washington, DC, 1
women: childbirth, 52; "empowered," 82; invisibility, 49–50; maternal mortality, 7, 9, 11, 18, 27–28, 41–44, 51; partner violence against, 10, 14; physicians, 45; rape, 10
World Food Programme (2003), 120
World Health Organization (WHO): cancer program, 156, 174, 181; conceptions of health, 232; death estimates, 6; on Iraq, 117, 121, 141; on Pakistan, 62; polio, 57, 64, 66, 90–91; on radiation, 181
World Trade Center, 92

Yemen, 137, 154, 173